Intravenous

Therapy

for Prehospital Providers

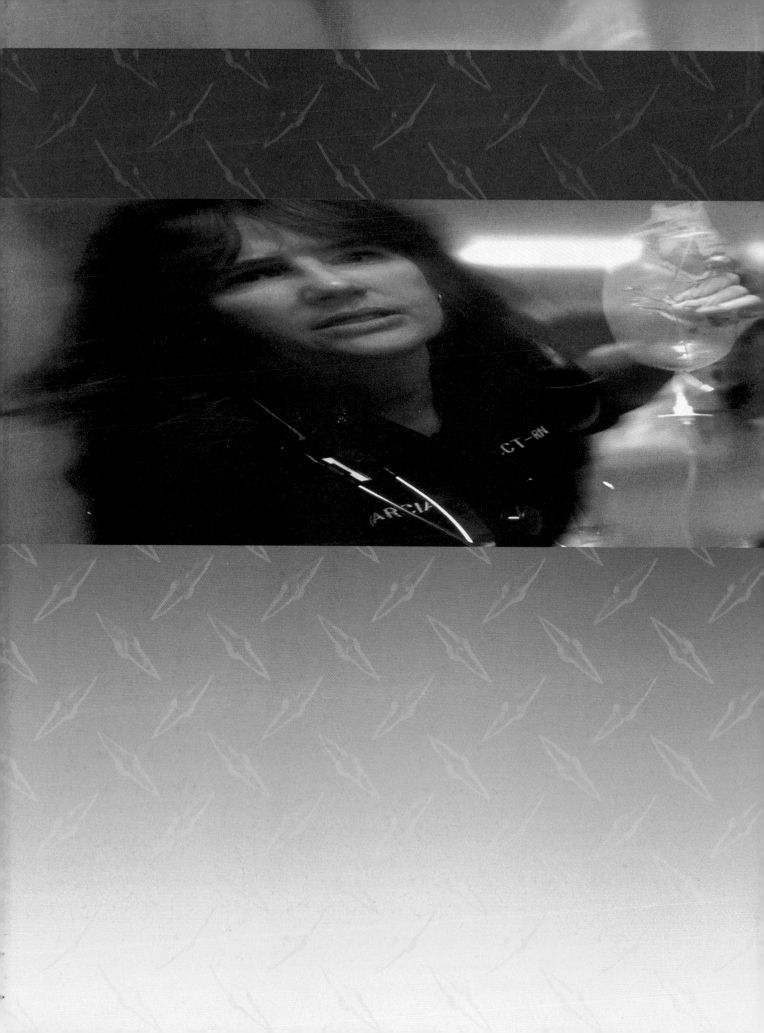

Intravenous

Therapy

for Prehospital Providers

American Academy of Orthopaedic Surgeons

Author:

Christopher M. Andolsek

JONES AND BARTLETT PUBLISHERS

Sudbury, Massachusetts

BOSTON   TORONTO   LONDON   SINGAPORE

Jones and Bartlett Publishers

40 Tall Pine Drive
Sudbury, MA 01776
978-443-5000
info@jbpub.com
www.jbpub.com

Jones and Bartlett Publishers Canada

2406 Nikanna Road
Mississauga, ON L5C 2W6
CANADA

Jones and Bartlett Publishers International

Barb House, Barb Mews
London W6 7PA
UK

Production Credits

Emergency Care Editor: Kimberly Brophy
Associate Editor: Carol Brewer
Senior Production Editor: Linda DeBruyn
Production/Editorial Assistant: Janna Wasilewski
V.P. Manufacturing and Inventory Control: Therese Bräuer
Design and Composition: Studio Montage
Cover: Studio Montage
Cover Photograph: © Paul Kuroda/SuperStock, Inc.
Cover Printing: Lehigh Press
Text Printing and Binding: Courier Corporation
Web Design: Kristin Ohlin

American Academy of Orthopaedic Surgeons

Vice President, Education Programs: Mark W. Wieting
Director, Department of Publications: Marilyn L. Fox, PhD
Managing Editor: Lynne Roby Shindoll
Senior Editor: Barbara A. Scotese

This textbook is intended solely as a guide to the appropriate procedures to be employed when rendering emergency care to the sick and injured. It is not intended as a statement of the standards of care required in any particular situation, because circumstances and the patient's physical condition can vary widely from one emergency to another. Nor is it intended that this textbook shall in any way advise emergency personnel concerning legal authority to perform the activities or procedures discussed. Such local determinations should be made only with the aid of legal counsel.

Library of Congress Cataloging-in-Publication Data

Andolsek, Christopher M.
　　Intravenous therapy for prehospital providers / American Academy of Orthopaedic Surgeons; author, Christopher M. Andolsek.
　　　　p.;　cm.
　　ISBN 0-7637-1579-4
　　1. Intravenous therapy. 2. Emergency medical technicians. I. American Academy of Orthopaedic Surgeons. II. Title.
　　[DNLM: 1. Infusions, Intravenous—methods. 2. Emergency Medical Technicians. 3. Infection Control. 4. Pharmaceutical Preparations—administration & dosage. 5. Shock—drug therapy. 6. Water-Electrolyte Balance. WB 354 A552i 2001]
　　RM170 .A49 2001
　　615'.6—dc21

for Library of Congress

2001029192
CIP

Additional credits appear on page 150 which constitutes a continuation of the copyright page.

Printed in the United States of America
05 04 03 02　　　　　　　　　　　　10 9 8 7 6 5 4 3 2

Contents

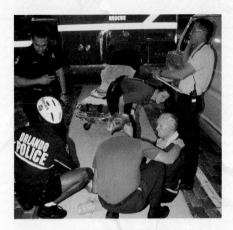

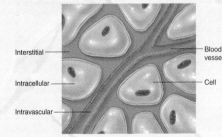

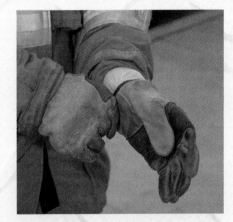

Interstitial — Blood vessel

Intracellular — Cell

Intravascular

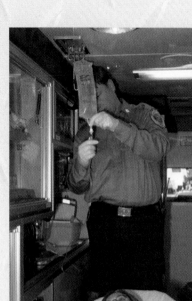

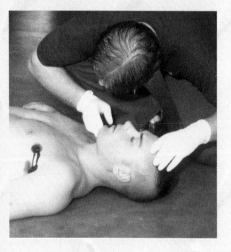

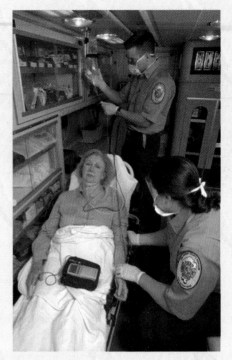

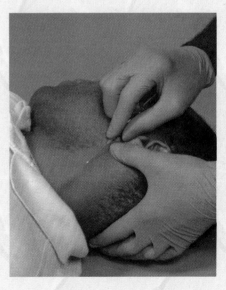

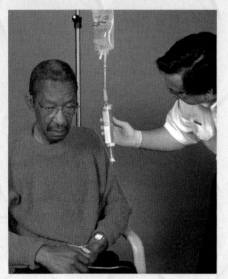

Acknowledgments

Jones & Bartlett Publishers and the author would like to thank the following people for reviewing this text.

Justin Bentzinger, RN, CEN, EMT-P, CRT
Director of Education
TerraMed International, Inc.
Wheat Ridge, CO

Mike Coakley
Alabama Fire College
Shelton State Community College
Tuscaloosa, AL

Dominic Foster, EMT-I
Genesys Regional Medical Center
Grand Blanc, MI

Michael K. Gammill, NREMT-P
Loudoun County Fire and Rescue Academy
Loudoun County, VA

James Levi, BS, NREMT-P
EHS Faculty
Inver Hills Community College
Inver Grove Heights, MN

Steve Moffitt
Alabama Fire College
Shelton State Community College
Tuscaloosa, AL

Lawrence D. Newell, Ed.D., NREMT-P
Educational Consultant, National Safety Council
Ashburn, VA

Jose V. Salazar, MPH, NREMT-P
President
Jose Salazar & Associates
Sterling, VA

Steve Sherrard, EMT-P, EMSIC, FF
Programs/Clinical Coordinator
Superior Medical Education
Madison Heights, MI

Daniel L. Sponsler
Division Chair
Program Director - Paramedicine A.A.S.
Northwest Technical College
East Grand Forks, MN

Technical and Photographic Consultants

Jim Brown
Maryland Institute for Emergency Medical
   Services Systems

Brian Slack
Maryland Institute for Emergency Medical
   Services Systems

William Seifarth, MS, NREMT-P
Maryland Institute for Emergency Medical
   Services Systems

Author Dedication

To my always vigilant and patient wife Jackie, thanks Mow!

Walk-Through

Intravenous Therapy for Prehospital Providers is written to teach prehospital personnel about IV therapy. It can be used in an IV therapy training course, or as a supplement in a course that teaches IV therapy along with other subjects.

Important topics include principles of fluid balance, IV techniques and administration, infection control, causes and treatment of shock, and altered level of consciousness. A section on practice calculations explains step-by-step how to calculate IV fluid dosage.

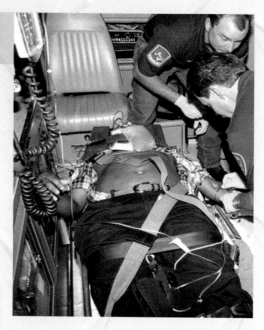

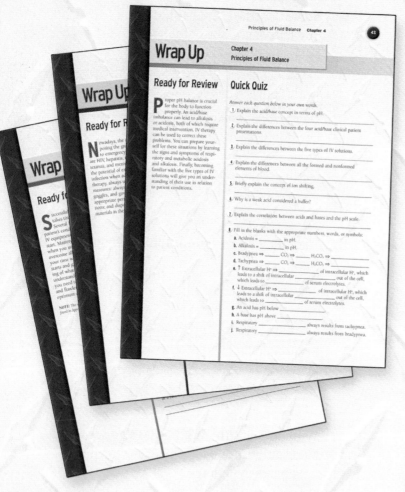

Special Features

- Contains a complete chapter on IV techniques and administration.
- A thorough chapter on principles of fluid balance familiarizes students with IV therapy's effects on the body.
- Separate chapters cover the role of IV therapy in treating shock and altered levels of consciousness.
- Dosage calculations are explained, then reinforced with practice calculations.
- Pediatric and geriatric considerations in IV therapy are covered in their own chapter.
- An IV Skills sheet is provided for self-testing. IV Starts Log sheets are provided for lab and field use.

Chapter Review

End-of-chapter questions allow students to test their knowledge of concepts presented in the chapter.

www.IVtherapy.EMSzone.com

Online resources are available at **www.IVtherapy.EMSzone.com**. Go to this site to test your knowledge of key terms, read online articles for extended coverage, and more.

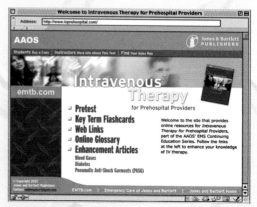

Introduction to IV Therapy:
Roles, Responsibilities, and Legal Issues

I ntravenous (IV) therapy is one of the most invasive procedures an EMT learns. During your career in Emergency Medical Services (EMS), few procedures will require more training or practice. Proficiency in IV therapy and technique is required for most procedures administered in advanced life support (**Figure 1-1**).

A medical problem of any type alters an individual's established balance among the systems of the body. This balance, called **homeostasis**, produces optimal physical performance. It is the job of health care providers to fully assess a patient and to find and treat life-threatening injuries and illnesses that alter homeostasis. Emergency Medical Technicians (EMTs) are often first on the scene and provide the first line of defense for individuals who need to have their homeostatic balance restored.

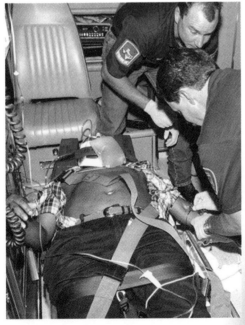

Figure 1-1 During your career in EMS, few procedures will require more training or practice than IV therapy.

> **I**V therapy is one of the most invasive procedures an EMT learns.

EMT Ethics and Responsibilities

As an EMT, you should be aware of the rules, roles, and responsibilities expected of you in the field. Working in EMS requires a new appreciation of legal obligations and responsibilities. Many allied health organizations have adopted oaths that define their roles in relationship to others and themselves. Just as doctors have the Hippocratic oath, EMTs have the EMT oath, which is shown in **Box 1-1**.

As a health care professional, you are expected to function in an honorable manner when dealing with patients, coworkers, and bystanders. These expectations are called ethics and are defined as a set of rules or standards of conduct designed by a group in order to govern that group. The medical community has had a code of ethics since the ancient Greek era. However, a code of ethics has no power if it is not honored. You are expected to act in an ethical, professional manner at all times, even when this is difficult. The National Association of Emergency Medical Technicians has created a code of ethics for the EMT community, including EMTs at the basic (EMT-B), intermediate (EMT-I), and paramedic (EMT-P) levels. This code of ethics is reproduced in **Box 1-2**.

Box 1-1: **The EMT Oath**

Be it pledged as an Emergency Medical Technician, I will honor the physical and judicial laws of God and man. I will follow that regimen which, according to my ability and judgment, I consider for the benefit of patients and abstain from whatever is deleterious and mischievous, nor shall I suggest any such counsel. Into whatever homes I enter, I will go into them for the benefit of only the sick and injured, never revealing what I see or hear in the lives of men unless required by law.

I shall also share my medical knowledge with those who may benefit from what I have learned. I will serve unselfishly and continuously in order to help make a better world for mankind.

While I continue to keep this oath unviolated, may it be granted to me to enjoy life, and the practice of the art, respected by all men, in all times. Should I trespass or violate this oath, may the reverse be my lot. So help me God.

National Association of Emergency Medical Technicians, 1978

Box 1-2:   EMT Code of Ethics

Professional status as an Emergency Medical Technician and EMT-P is maintained and enriched by the willingness of the individual practitioner to accept and fulfill obligations to society, other medical professionals, and the profession of the Emergency Medical Technician. As an Emergency Medical Technician at the Basic level or an Emergency Medical Technician-Paramedic, I solemnly pledge myself to the following code of professional ethics:

A fundamental responsibility of the Emergency Medical Technician is to conserve life, to alleviate suffering, to promote health, to do no harm, and to encourage the quality and equal availability of emergency medical care.

The Emergency Medical Technician provides services based on human need, with respect for human dignity, unrestricted by consideration of nationality, race, creed, color, or status.

The Emergency Medical Technician does not use professional knowledge and skills in any enterprise detrimental to the public well-being.

The Emergency Medical Technician respects and holds in confidence all information of a confidential nature obtained in the course of professional work unless required by law to divulge such information.

The Emergency Medical Technician, as a citizen, understands and upholds the law and performs the duties of citizenship; as a professional, the Emergency Medical Technician has the never-ending responsibility to work with concerned citizens and other health care professionals in promoting a high standard of emergency medical care to all people.

The Emergency Medical Technician shall maintain professional competence and demonstrate concern for the competence of other members of the Emergency Medical Services health care team.

An Emergency Medical Technician assumes responsibility in defining and upholding standards of professional practice and education.

The Emergency Medical Technician assumes responsibility for individual professional actions and judgment, both in dependent and independent emergency functions, and knows and upholds the laws which affect the practice of the Emergency Medical Technician.

An Emergency Medical Technician has the responsibility to be aware of and participate in matters of legislation affecting the Emergency Medical Service System.

The Emergency Medical Technician, or groups of Emergency Medical Technicians, who advertise professional service, do so in conformity with the dignity of the profession.

The Emergency Medical Technician has an obligation to protect the public by not delegating to a person less qualified any service which requires the professional competence of an Emergency Medical Technician.

The Emergency Medical Technician will work harmoniously with and sustain confidence in Emergency Medical Technician associates, the nurses, the physicians, and other members of the Emergency Medical Services health care team.

The Emergency Medical Technician refuses to participate in unethical procedures, and assumes the responsibility to expose incompetence or unethical conduct of others to the appropriate authority in a proper and professional manner.

Written by Charles Gillespie, MD

Adopted by the National Association of Emergency Medical Technicians, 1978

Professionalism

As an EMT, you must act professionally at all times. Being a professional takes dedication, constant training, and education to provide the best care for a patient. Continuing education keeps you up to date and comes in many different forms:

- Training provided by agencies
- Professional journals
- National and state conferences
- College courses

Part of being professional is knowing what your limitations are. The EMT must often decide what level of care the patient requires and how much he or she can provide. An EMT needs to have a clear understanding of his or her scope of practice, physician advisor guidelines, and agency standing orders and protocols.

Professionalism is more of an attitude than a function. Professionals generally take great pride in their work—even when they do not receive recognition or praise from others.

Leadership

The EMT at any level of training is often looked upon as a leader—someone who can take charge of a situation and maintain the focus of the team to accomplish a goal (**Figure 1-2**). Throughout history, certain characteristics have defined the qualities of a leader:

- An ability to remain calm and in control that instills confidence in others
- Inner strength to make a decision and live with the consequences of that decision
- Solid character traits that inspire trust among others
- Solid moral and ethical beliefs
- The ability to communicate

Figure 1-2 The EMT as a leader.

Acts Allowed

In most states, the acts you are allowed to perform are clearly defined by your state EMS regulatory agency and physician advisory. The **acts allowed**, which defines your scope of practice, lists the skills and drugs that you are authorized to use. For example, in Colorado, the acts allowed for EMT-Bs include:

- Performing noninvasive emergency medical treatment as outlined by the state EMS division
- Inflating **pneumatic anti-shock garments (PASG)** and inserting **peripheral IVs** for volume replacement or dextrose administration

acts allowed
The tasks that an EMT is allowed to perform, as defined by the state EMS regulatory agency and physician advisory.

- Using an **automated external defibrillator (AED)** in accordance with the training outlined in the U.S. Department of Transportation EMT–Basic National Standard Curriculum

Standard of Care

EMTs at any level of training are expected to provide a uniform level of patient care across the country. This level of care is called the **standard of care**. It reflects a minimally accepted level of care that should be provided by any EMS care provider around the country. Your failure to meet these minimally accepted levels of care could place you at risk of legal repercussions.

standard of care
A uniform level of care that EMTs are expected to provide to all patients.

Legal Issues for the EMT

Every person has, and is entitled to, certain legal rights. As an EMT, you have the right to protection from abusive patients and dangerous situations. Your patient also has certain legal rights, which you cannot violate. You can be held legally accountable for the following actions:

- **False imprisonment:** The illegal detention of a patient against his or her will when transporting the person to the hospital.

- **Torts:** Civil wrongs that can end in lawsuits even if no criminal act was committed.

- **Assault:** The threat of injury directed at either the patient or the EMT.

- **Battery:** The physical contact that occurs illegally between an EMT and the patient unless the patient has given permission for treatment.

- **Negligence:** Deviation from the accepted standard of care that results in further injury to the patient.

- **Abandonment:** The termination of patient care without assuring that care will be continued at the same medical level or higher. When administering IV therapy, you have the obligation to ensure that someone who has at least the same certification level as yourself will continue patient care. Remember, once patient contact has been established, you are legally bound to remain with your patient until one of the following criteria is met:

  - You hand over care to someone as equally certified as you.

  - The patient terminates care after meeting the required criteria for competency.

  Patient abandonment does not apply if your safety is at risk. In that case, your first responsibility is to yourself and your EMS partners.

> **T**he EMT must often decide what level of care the patient requires and how much he or she can provide.

> **N**egligence can be established if further injury to the patient resulted from a deviation from the accepted standard of care.

Negligence

Malfeasance

Malfeasance is defined as wrongdoing that is illegal or contrary to official obligations. Negligence can be established if there is deviation from the accepted standard of care that results in further injury to the patient. To establish negligence, certain criteria must be met:

- There must be a duty to act for the EMT in the first place. While employed and on the clock for an EMS agency, EMS personnel have a duty to act.
- The EMT breeched that duty to act.

Nonfeasance

Nonfeasance is defined as a failure to perform some act that is either an official duty or a legal requirement. An example would be not performing CPR when you witness a **cardiac arrest.** In such a case, the failure of the EMT to act could cause injury to the patient.

Misfeasance

Misfeasance is defined as the improper and unlawful execution of some act that itself is lawful and proper. For example, an EMT who chose to apply a skill that was beyond his or her level of training, such as inappropriate administration of a medication, could be accused of misfeasance if the patient dies.

Patient Refusals

If a patient refuses treatment, you should obtain a release waiver. Obtaining a **patient refusal waiver** requires caution; you must be sure that the patient understands why he or she is refusing treatment, exactly what he or she is refusing, and what the consequences of refusal are. It is not as simple as getting a signature. If a patient's refusal of treatment ever becomes involved in litigation, you must be able to prove that the patient understood the consequences of his or her actions.

Some considerations that could affect the patient's ability to understand the consequences of refusing treatment include:

- Substance abuse
- Language
- Injury or illness
- Shock

Below are some simple rules to follow if a patient refuses treatment and you need to obtain a waiver:

1. Explain the mechanism of injury and your concern for the patient's well-being.
2. Have the patient state his or her interpretation of what you said about the condition.
3. Explain that you want to do a patient assessment to assure both of you that the injuries or illnesses are not life threatening.

RELEASE FROM RESPONSIBILITY WHEN PATIENT REFUSES IV THERAPY

This is to certify that I, _____, am refusing IV treatment. I acknowledge
patient's name

that I have been informed of the risk involved and hereby release the emergency medical services

provider(s), the physician consultant, and the consulting hospital from all responsibility for any

ill effects which may result from this action.

Witness _____   Signed _____
                                                          patient name or nearest relative

Witness _____   _____
                                                          relationship

---

RELEASE FROM RESPONSIBILITY WHEN PATIENT REFUSES SERVICE

This is to certify that I, _____, am refusing the services offered by the
patient's name

emergency medical services provider(s). I acknowledge that I have been informed of the risk

involved and hereby release the emergency medical services provider(s), the physician consultant,

and the consulting hospital from all responsibility for any ill effects which may result from this action.

Witness _____   Signed _____
                                                          patient name or nearest relative

Witness _____   _____
                                                          relationship

---

RELEASE FROM RESPONSIBILITY WHEN PATIENT REFUSES SERVICES
BUT ACCEPTS TRANSPORT

This is to certify that I, _____, am refusing _____
patient's name

_____. I acknowledge that I have been informed of the risk involved

and hereby release the emergency medical services provider(s), the physician consultant, and the

consulting hospital from all responsibility for any ill effects which may result from this action.

However, I do accept transportation to a medical facility.

Witness _____   Signed _____
                                                          patient name or nearest relative

Witness _____   _____
                                                          relationship

Figure 1-3 Refusal form.

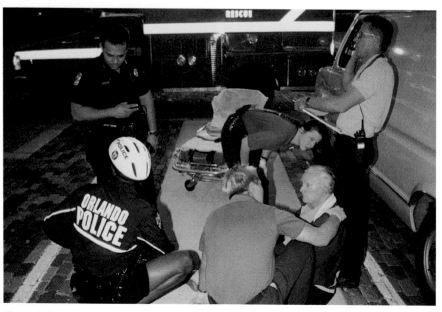

Figure 1-4 In obtaining a patient refusal, you must be sure the patient understands the consequences of refusing treatment.

SAMPLE history
A key brief history of a patient's condition to determine Signs/symptoms, Allergies, Medications, Pertinent past history, Last oral intake, and Events leading to the illness/injury.

4. To ensure that there are no additional life-threatening injuries, check vital signs, physically examine the patient, and obtain a **SAMPLE history.**

5. Obtain the patient's signature on the patient refusal form, acknowledging findings and refusal.

6. Attempt to obtain a signature from a witness.

7. Document the patient's explanation for refusing treatment.

Advance Directives

An **advance directive** is defined as an agreement between a patient and a physician indicating a course of action to be taken should the patient become incompetent. Advance directives are becoming more common among terminally ill patients. You are expected to honor and execute the wishes of the patient when you encounter advance directives. Some advance directives are legally binding documents, and failure to honor these documents can place you at risk of criminal litigation.

Do Not Resuscitate Orders

When faced with a DNR, it is crucial to ensure that it is accurate and authentic.

Do not resuscitate (DNR) orders specifically identify the medical procedures to be performed on the patient in the event of cardiac arrest. DNR orders are rescindable only by verbal order of the patient or legal guardian, physician, or immediate family member, or by physical destruction of the document.

To be considered valid, a DNR order must meet specific criteria. The document must be specific to the patient and the underlying medical condition. Information that must be presented with a DNR order includes:

1. Name of the patient

2. Reason for the DNR order

3. Name and signature of the responsible physician

4. Date on which the order became effective

5. DNR or Do Not Resuscitate wording

6. Patient consent, evidenced by one of the following:

   • Patient's signature

   • Signature of legal guardian

   • Signature of holder of durable medical power of attorney

When faced with a DNR order, you must validate the order by verifying that it is accurate and authentic. The DNR order must be for the patient for whom you are caring. You must also validate the patient's name, the signature, and the DNR effective date. If the DNR order is accurate, it must be honored and executed. If a declarant indicates that he or she wishes to revoke the DNR at any time, this request must be honored. If you have any concerns about the validity of the document, you must contact medical control while resuscitative measures are initiated. If medical control directs you to cease resuscitative efforts, you are required to comply.

Durable Medical Power of Attorney

A **durable medical power of attorney** is a document that directs someone to act on behalf of the patient regarding medical treatment. These documents are often used for patients who are incapacitated in some fashion. A durable medical power of attorney is often granted to a legal guardian acting as an agent for the patient's medical concerns. The agent must act on behalf of the patient, not on the agent's own behalf. If the patient is **competent** and requests treatment other than what is listed in the durable medical power of attorney, the request must be honored despite the wishes of the agent or the document. The durable medical power of attorney is revocable by a competent patient at any time. When faced with a durable medical power of attorney, you should:

   • Ensure it is valid.

   • Verify the identity of the agent.

   • Make sure the agent is acting in the patient's best interest.

   • Check the patient's mental status.

If there is any doubt about the validity of the document, contact medical control.

> **I**f the patient is competent and requests treatment other than what is listed in the durable medical power of attorney, the request must be honored.

Living Wills

A **living will** is a legal document completed by a competent patient who has not developed any medical disorders that expresses the patient's wishes regarding medical treatment should he or she become incompetent. For example, a living will would come into play when a patient enters a hospital for surgery or some other potentially dangerous medical procedure. Therefore, living wills are seldom encountered in the field. As with acts allowed and protocols, check your state's regulation on advance directives and living wills.

Wrap Up

Chapter 1
Introduction to IV Therapy:
Roles, Responsibilities, and Legal Issues

Ready for Review

By understanding the EMT's legal and ethical responsibilities, you will gain a solid foundation for providing safe IV therapy. The following steps will help you achieve this goal:

- Study your local protocols and acts allowed.

- Know the actions that can lead to legal accountability: false imprisonment, torts, assault, battery, negligence, and abandonment.

- Understand what is meant by negligence: deviation from the accepted standard of care resulting in further injury to the patient when the EMT has a duty to act but does not.

- When dealing with patient refusals, ensure that the patient understands the consequences of refusal and document the refusal.

- When dealing with advance directives, DNRs, and durable medical power of attorney documents, ensure that the document is valid.

Quick Quiz

Answer each question below in your own words.

1. List and describe each component required to establish negligence of the rescuer.

2. Describe patient abandonment. When is it acceptable to leave a patient?

3. What is meant by standard of care?

4. List and describe the different forms of advance directives.

5. What are some barriers that you need to be aware of when obtaining a patient refusal?

6. List the steps you should follow before accepting a patient treatment refusal.

7. List and describe the legal issues for which you may be held accountable as an EMT.

Infection Control

Protection from infectious diseases is a major concern for the EMS community. With drug-resistant strains of diseases becoming more common, the primary focus must be on preventing exposure to **infection,** rather than treating infection after exposure has occurred.

Body Substance Isolation

Exposure to disease can be minimized by practicing **body substance isolation (BSI).** If you have patient contact, you must be aware of the possibility of exposure to infectious body fluids and must take the necessary precautions. Ultimately, the responsibility for your personal safety rests your hands. If you ignore the importance of personal protection, you place yourself and others at extreme risk. BSI protection includes several components that together help prevent exposure to infection: gloves, gowns, goggles, personal immunization, and proper disposal of contaminated items.

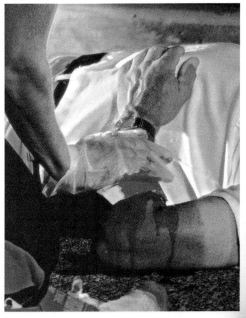

Gloves

You should wear latex or vinyl gloves during all patient contact. If used correctly, gloves will protect you from contact with body fluids (**Figure 2-1**). Correct procedure can be difficult to remember and follow, but if you practice the following steps early in your career, they will become second nature.

Figure 2-1 Gloves must be worn during all patient contact.

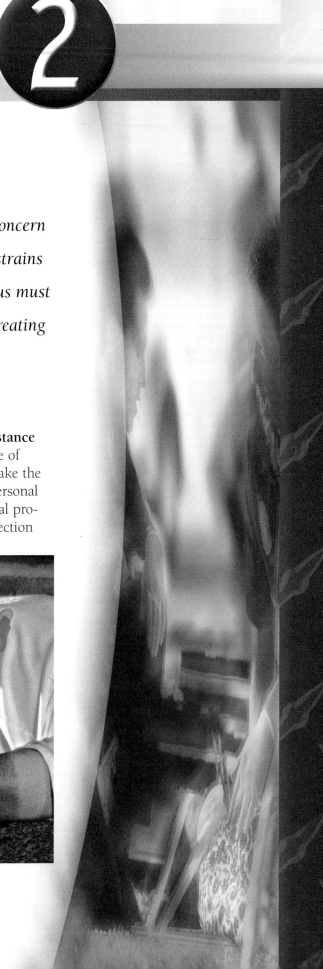

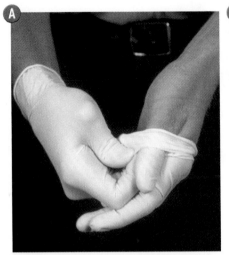
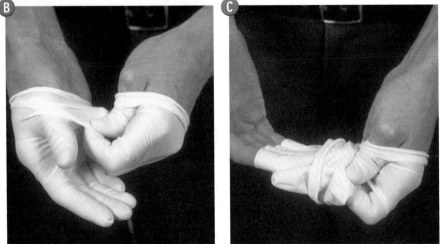
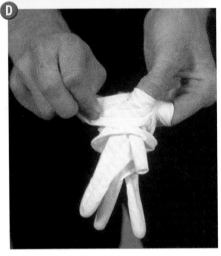

Figure 2-2   Proper technique for removal of gloves.   **A.** Partially remove the first glove by pinching at the wrist. Be careful to touch only the outside of the glove.   **B.** Remove the second glove by pinching the exterior with the partially gloved hand.   **C.** Pull the second glove inside out toward the fingertips.   **D.** Grasp both gloves with your free hand touching only the clean, interior surfaces.

1. Always wear gloves during patient contact. If you need to leave your patient, remove your gloves before you touch any other item. When you return, put on a new pair of gloves—this will help prevent **cross-contamination** of equipment and other personnel.

2. Begin by partially removing one glove. With the other gloved hand, pinch the first glove at the wrist—being certain to *touch only the outside* of the first glove—and start to roll it back off the hand, inside out. Leave the exterior of the fingers on that first glove exposed. Use the still-gloved fingers of the first hand to pinch the wrist of the second glove and begin to pull it off, rolling it inside-out toward the fingertips as you did with the first glove. Continue pulling the second glove off until you can pull that second hand free. With your now-ungloved second hand, grasp the exposed *inside* of the first glove and pull it free of your first hand and over the now-loose second glove. Be sure that you touch only clean, interior surfaces with your ungloved hand (**Figure 2-2**).

3. Immediately dispose of contaminated gloves in a properly identified medical waste container.

4. Wash your hands as soon as possible after removing your gloves to eliminate any microscopic contamination. Cuticles and skin folds can hide bacteria that can be a cause for concern. Use anti-microbial soap if possible.

5. Soap can seriously dry the skin of your hands, causing them to crack and bleed. Use a good hand lotion after washing to ensure skin integrity, thus adding to your protection from infection.

6. If you are involved in an **extrication** procedure, heavy gloves are a must, as latex or vinyl gloves will easily tear (**Figure 2-3**). Fire department approved gloves contain a moisture barrier that will prevent fluid from cross-contaminating. If you are not sure whether the type of heavy gloves you are using contains this barrier, wear a pair of latex or vinyl gloves under the heavier gloves.

extrication
Removal of a patient from entrapment or a dangerous situation or position, such as removal from a wrecked vehicle, industrial accident, or building collapse.

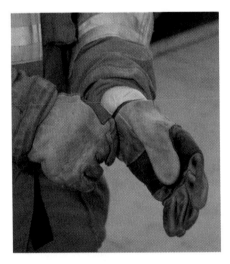

Figure 2-3 If you might be involved in extrication procedures, heavy gloves are a must.

Gowns

Often overlooked, disposable paper gowns are ideal for protection from heavily contaminated patients. Patients who are covered with blood or chemicals, or who have **systemic** infections can contaminate your uniform without your being aware of the exposure. As with gloves, you must use gowns correctly:

1. Wear the gown during patient contact.

2. Remove the gown immediately after patient treatment to avoid the possibility of accidentally cross-contaminating yourself, the rig, or your equipment.

3. Immediately dispose of the contaminated gown. Be aware of the type of disposal you need, because some exposures require **HazMat containment.**

4. If you are involved in a heavy extrication procedure, **bunker gear** serves as a good body fluid barrier because it contains a moisture barrier (**Figure 2-4**). Cleanup of bunker gear can be problematic if you do not have access to proper storage and cleaning equipment. Rewearing contaminated bunker gear is like reusing contaminated gloves on another patient—you may expose others to potential hazards.

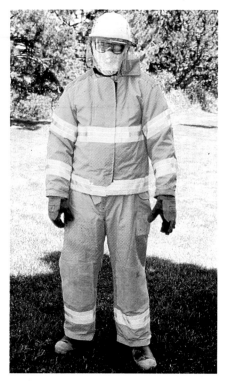

Figure 2-4 Bunker gear is a good fluid barrier for heavy extrication procedures.

Goggles

You should wear safety goggles whenever body fluid splashing or spraying is a possibility (**Figure 2-5**). Eyeglasses are better than nothing, but safety goggles protect from the sides as well as from the front. Safety goggles *must* be used in heavy extrications.

Infectious Diseases

Serious infection is possible whenever you come into contact with any contaminated material or substance. Diseases can be transmitted in various ways, including casual contact, airborne transmission, and bloodborne transmission. Most transmittable diseases are nothing more than inconveniences (such as a cold), but some can be very serious.

HIV and AIDS

The **human immunodeficiency virus (HIV)** is the precursor to **acquired immunodeficiency syndrome (AIDS).** The virus is transmitted when infected blood comes in contact with uninfected blood through actual blood contact or through contact with blood-rich **mucous membranes.** HIV destroys the immune system by infecting and turning off the **T-cells** of the immune system, effectively shutting down the ability of the immune system to recognize and destroy foreign invaders. Once a person has been exposed to the virus, HIV can lie dormant and undetectable for up to a year. After detection, HIV can take several years before infecting the immune system.

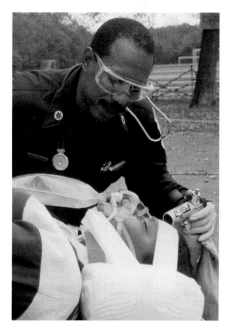

Figure 2-5 Wear safety goggles when splashing of body fluids is a possibility.

Hepatitis

Hepatitis is a viral disease characterized by infection and inflammation of the liver. Hepatitis actually includes several different viral diseases, each of which is contracted in its own way and progresses on its own course. The courses for hepatitis A, B, and C, are described below. All types of hepatitis can lead to permanent damage of the liver. Hepatitis is also spread throughout the rest of the body by blood circulation; people infected with hepatitis, especially hepatitis B and hepatitis C, are therefore not considered good candidates for liver transplants because the infection will return to the new liver.

Health care workers are among those at risk for infection with hepatitis B and C. The American Liver Foundation's informational booklet *Getting Hip to Hep—What You Should Know About Hepatitis A, B, & C* defines and describes the three types of hepatitis as follows:

- Hepatitis A virus (HAV) is contracted by eating food or drinking water that has been contaminated with human feces. Symptoms usually appear 15 to 45 days following exposure to the infection. Acute hepatitis A usually resolves itself within 6 months and does not develop into a chronic disease. Vaccination is the best prevention against hepatitis A.

- Hepatitis B virus (HBV) can cause a serious form of hepatitis. This disease is much more prevalent than HIV, the AIDS virus. The hepatitis B virus transmission is from bodily fluid exposure, which includes blood, semen and saliva. Symptoms usually appear within 25 to 180 days following exposure. Hepatitis B may develop into a chronic disease (lasting more than 6 months) in up to 10% of the 140,000 to 320,000 newly infected people each year. The risk of developing **cirrhosis** (scarring of the liver) and liver cancer is increased in untreated patients with chronic HBV. Vaccination is the best protection against hepatitis.

- Hepatitis C virus (HCV) is transmitted by exposure to an infected person's blood. The onset of the infection is often unrecognized and that is why it is often described as the "quiet virus." Some people may experience fatigue, loss of appetite and/or nausea. Hepatitis C develops into a chronic infection in up to 85% of the 36,000 newly infected people each year. Like chronic hepatitis B, if left untreated, the chronic form of hepatitis C has a greater chance of developing into cirrhosis, liver cancer, or even liver failure. There is no vaccine available.

Tuberculosis

Once only a briefly mentioned respiratory disease in most emergency medicine texts, **tuberculosis (TB)** is now a more commonly seen medical problem. Although TB is considered to be a disease of poor populations, it is also a front-line threat to EMS personnel. TB is most often seen in homeless, drug abuse, and immigrant populations, as well as in **immunocompromised** patients, such as HIV-infected individuals. Because TB is an airborne disease, you should be fitted with a **HEPAmask** designed to prevent inhalation of the tuberculosis bacterium (**Figure 2-6**). Control should also include masking the patient.

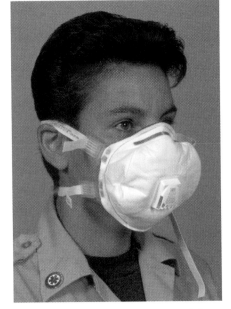

Figure 2-6 HEPAmasks prevent the inhalation of the tuberculosis bacterium.

> **M**eningitis occurs in populations
> that live in close proximity and are unlikely to have access
> to immediate health care.

Tetanus

Tetanus, also called lockjaw, is a rapidly developing infection that targets the central nervous system. The main cause of this disease is the toxin produced by *Clostridium tetani,* a common bacterium found in soil or on anything that has come in contact with soil. Patients develop headache, irritability, fever, and, ultimately, painful muscle spasms that become continuous muscle contractions.

Meningitis

Meningitis is an infection of the meninges, the membranes surrounding the brain and spinal cord. The infection is spread by the circulating cerebrospinal fluid (CSF). Meningitis can be passed to others who come into contact with contaminated body fluids or who breathe in the bacteria expelled from the lungs by coughing. Meningitis infections tend to occur in populations that live in confined or close quarters, such as prisons, college dorms, nursing homes, or multi-family households. Neonates, children, and people without access to immediate health care are also at risk.

Personal Immunizations

One of the best ways to protect yourself from infection is to obtain all of the appropriate tests and immunizations.

- Complete the hepatitis B series. This is a one-time immunization series, but you should get a booster shot every 10 years.

- Have a TB skin test done annually, or every 6 months if you are in a high-risk environment. Get a chest X-ray after a positive skin test.

- Tetanus/diphtheria toxoid is a very effective preventive **inoculant** that protects against both tetanus and **diphtheria**. Booster shots should be given every 5 to 10 years.

- Take Hib (*Haemophilus influenzae* type B) inoculations to help prevent *Haemophilus influenzae* infections.

- Annual influenza injections are not a bad idea. These injections are proving very reliable in prevention of the illness.

- Consider an inoculant against bacterial forms of pneumonia. The period of protection is similar in length to the tetanus injection—about 5 to 10 years.

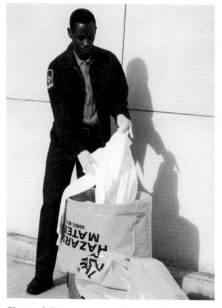

Figure 2-7 Contaminated linens, patient clothing, and call-related trash are all disposed of in large biohazard bags.

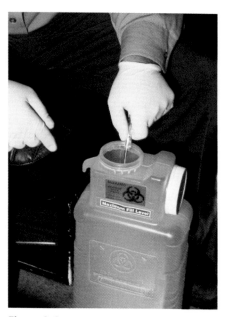

Figure 2-8 Always dispose of sharp objects or blood-filled items in a sharps container.

Disposal of Contaminated Items

After items have been contaminated with body fluids, correct disposal is critical. **Biohazard bags** are used to contain contaminated items. All biohazard containers are colored red for rapid identification. These containers are intended for contaminated items only and should not be used as convenient trash cans. Different items require various levels of handling:

1. Dispose of contaminated linens, patient clothing, and call-related trash (bloody gloves, soaked gauze, etc.) in large biohazard bags (**Figure 2-7**).

2. Dispose of any sharp objects or blood-filled containers (blood tubes, syringes) in hard plastic **sharps containers** (**Figure 2-8**). These containers are puncture- and crush-resistant. *Never* attempt to retrieve any item dropped into a sharps container.

3. Take contaminated equipment out of service until it is cleaned and cleared to be used again. Such equipment may include:

    a. Contaminated crew clothing (personal clothing, bunker gear)

    b. Contaminated ambulance equipment (anything that has come in contact with patient body fluids)

    c. A contaminated ambulance resulting from environmental exposure (toxic chemicals, for example, spread by a patient who suffered full exposure to such chemicals) or serious disease exposure (patient blood, patient body fluids, or airborne diseases)

Wrap Up

**Chapter 2
Infection Control**

Ready for Review

Nowadays, the infections posing the greatest threat to emergency personnel are HIV, hepatitis, tuberculosis, tetanus, and meningitis. To reduce the potential of exposure to infection when administering IV therapy, always use BSI preventive measures: always wear gloves, goggles, and gowns; obtain all appropriate personal immunizations; and dispose of contaminated materials in their proper containers.

Quick Quiz

Answer each question below in your own words.

1. Discuss the different forms of hepatitis.

   _____

2. Discuss the different BSI items.

   _____

3. Discuss the differences between HIV and HBV.

   _____

4. Discuss the significance of tuberculosis exposure for EMS personnel.

   _____

5. Discuss the differences between the three types of hepatitis infections.

   _____

6. Describe the type of patient contact situations that might expose an EMT to the risk of meningitis infection.

   _____

7. Describe the type of patient contact situations that might expose an EMT to the risk of tuberculosis infection.

   _____

8. Describe the type of patient contact situations that might expose an EMT to the risk of hepatitis infection.

   _____

9. Discuss suggested personal immunizations, including the recommended frequency of injections.

   _____

10. Discuss the proper disposal method for items contaminated by body fluids.

   _____

Basic Cell Physiology

A human cell can exist only in a special balanced environment. Understanding how this environment is created and maintained will give you the foundation you need to perform IV therapy.

Because the cell is completely enclosed by a cell membrane, compounds must move through the membrane to enter the cell. Small compounds like water (H_2O), carbon dioxide (CO_2), hydrogen ions (H^+), and oxygen (O_2) can easily pass through the membrane. Larger charged compounds need assistance to cross the cell membrane and enter the cell.

The cell membrane is a selective barrier. It chooses which compounds to allow across, depending on the needs of the cell. This **selective permeability** of the cell membrane is due to its composition (**Figure 3-1**). The cell membrane is a **phospholipid bilayer**—that is, it has two parts:

- A **hydrophilic** outer layer made up of phosphate groups
- A **hydrophobic** inner layer made up of lipids or fatty acids

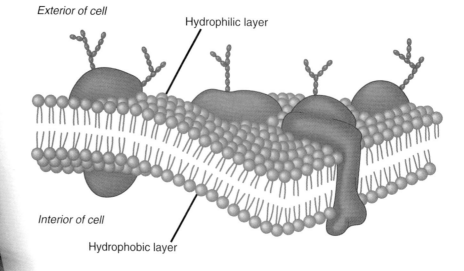

Exterior of cell

Hydrophilic layer

Interior of cell

Hydrophobic layer

Figure 3-1 The phospholipid bilayer.

This bilayer is a very important barrier to fluid movement and the acid/base balance, which will be covered in Chapter 4, "Principles of Fluid Balance." Everything discussed in this text will in some way be related to the cell membrane barrier and movement across it.

Electrolytes

Atoms carry charges—some positive, some negative. Two or more atoms that bond together form a molecule. When atoms bond together, they share and disperse their charges throughout the molecule. Molecules containing carbon atoms—for example, table sugar ($C_6H_{12}O_6$)—are called organic molecules. Molecules created without carbon—for example, table salt (NaCl)—are called inorganic molecules. Inorganic molecules give rise to **electrolytes** when they disassociate in water into their charged components. For example, table salt disassociates into sodium (Na^+) and chlorine (Cl^-).

Charged atoms and charged compounds are called electrolytes because of their ability to conduct electricity. Electrolytes, also called **ions,** are reactive and dangerous if left to circulate in the body, but the body uses the energy stored in these charged particles. Electrolytes help to regulate everything from water levels to cardiac function and muscle contractions. Water in the body helps to stabilize the electrolyte charges so that the electrolytes can be used to perform the **metabolic** functions that are necessary to life.

Each electrolyte has a unique property or value to the body and is used in a different way. If the electrolyte has an overall positive charge, it is called a **cation;** an electrolyte with an overall negative charge is called an **anion.** The major cations of the body include sodium, potassium, and calcium; bicarbonate and phosphate are the major anions.

Sodium

Sodium (Na^+) is the principal extracellular cation needed to regulate the distribution of water throughout the body in the **intravascular** and **interstitial** fluid compartments, making it a major factor in adequate **cellular perfusion.** This gives rise to the saying, "Where sodium goes, water follows." Sodium is also a major component of the circulating **buffer** sodium bicarbonate ($NaHCO_3$). (Buffers are discussed in Chapter 4, "Principles of Fluid Balance.")

Potassium

About 98% of all the body's potassium (K^+) is found inside the cells of the body, making it the principal intracellular cation. Potassium plays a major role in neuromuscular function as well as in the conversion of glucose into glycogen. Cellular potassium levels are regulated by insulin. The **sodium/potassium** (Na^+/K^+) **pump** (see "Fluid Compartments" on page 23) is helped by the presence of insulin and **epinephrine.** Low potassium levels—<u>hypokalemia</u>—in the serum (blood plasma) can lead to decreased skeletal muscle function, gastrointestinal (GI) disturbances, and alterations in cardiac function. High potassium levels in the serum—<u>hyperkalemia</u>—can lead to hyperstimulation of neural cell transmission, resulting in cardiac arrest.

> **O**ne unique feature of water in the body is that it helps to stabilize the charges of electrolytes so that the electrolytes can be used to perform metabolic functions that are necessary to life.

<u>hypokalemia</u>
Low levels of potassium.

<u>hyperkalemia</u>
High levels of potassium.

Calcium

Calcium (Ca^{2+}) is the principal cation needed for bone growth. It plays an important part in the functioning of heart muscle, nerves, and cell membranes and is necessary for proper blood clotting.

Low serum calcium levels—**hypocalcemia**—can lead to overstimulation of nerve cells, resulting in the following signs and symptoms:

- Skeletal muscle cramps
- Abdominal cramps
- **Carpal/pedal spasms**
- **Hypotension**
- **Vasoconstriction**

High serum calcium levels—**hypercalcemia**—can lead to decreased stimulation of nerve cells, resulting in the following signs and symptoms:

- Skeletal muscle weakness
- Lethargy
- **Ataxia**
- **Vasodilation**
- Hot, flushed skin

hypocalcemia
Low levels of serum calcium.

hypercalcemia
High levels of serum calcium.

Bicarbonate

Bicarbonate (HCO_3^-) levels are the determining factor between **acidosis** and **alkalosis** in the body. Sodium bicarbonate is the primary buffer used in all circulating body fluids.

Chloride

Chloride (Cl^-) primarily regulates the **pH** of the stomach. It also regulates extracellular fluid levels.

Phosphate

Phosphate (PO_4^{3-}) is an important component in the formation of adenosine triphosphate (ATP), the powerful energy supplier of the body.

Fluid and Electrolyte Movement

Water and electrolytes move among the body's fluid compartments (see "Fluid Compartments" on page 23) according to some basic chemical and biologic tenets. One of these governing principles is that unequal concentrations on different sides of a cell membrane will move to balance themselves equally on both sides of the membrane. Balance across a cell membrane has two components:

- Balance of compounds (water, electrolytes, etc.) on either side of the cell membrane
- Balance of charges (the + or - charges carried on the atoms) on either side of the cell membrane

When concentrations of charges or compounds are greater on one side of the cell membrane than on the other, a gradient is created.

The natural tendency for materials is to flow from an area of higher concentration to one of lower concentration. This movement establishes a <u>concentration gradient</u>. Gradients are categorized according to the type of material that flows down them; chemical compounds flow down chemical gradients; electrical currents flow down electrical gradients. The process of flowing down a gradient depends on whether the cell membrane will allow the material to pass through it. Certain compounds can travel freely across the cell membrane, a kinetically favorable situation that requires little energy, while others require active transport across the membrane, either because of the size of the compound or because of an incompatible charge.

<u>concentration gradient</u>
The natural tendency for substances to flow from an area of higher concentration to an area of lower concentration, either within the cell or outside the cell.

Diffusion

Compounds or charges concentrated on one side of a cell membrane will move across it to an area of lower concentration to balance themselves across the membrane, a process called **diffusion.** To visualize this, imagine that too many people show up for a theater performance. The management decides to open another seating area to accommodate the crowd. Patrons (charges or compounds) are concentrated in the small seating area (the cell) outside the door (the cell membrane) leading to the new seating area. When the theater manager opens the door, patrons can move through (selective cell membrane permeability) from the congested seating area (down a concentration gradient). The patrons spread themselves out evenly (diffuse) throughout the total area, some choosing to stay behind in the original seating area as others move into the new area, so that they all have an equal amount of room.

Filtration

Filtration is another type of diffusion, commonly used by the kidneys to clean blood. Water carries dissolved compounds across the cell membranes of the **tubules** of the kidney. The tubule membrane then traps these dissolved compounds but lets the water pass through, in much the same way that a coffee filter traps the grounds as water passes through it. This cleans the blood of wastes and removes the trapped compounds from circulation so they can be flushed out of the body. The **antidiuretic hormone (ADH)** prevents the loss of water from the kidneys by causing its reabsorption into the tubules. ADH plays an important role in **diabetes insipidus.**

Active Transport

Often, the cell must maintain an imbalance of compounds across its membrane to achieve some metabolic purpose. An example of such an imbalance is the sodium/potassium pump. The cell uses sodium outside the cell and potassium inside the cell for an important cellular function called **depolarization.** To maintain this imbalance, the cell must use energy in the form of ATP and actively transport compounds across its membrane. Even though active transport demands a high energy expenditure, the benefits outweigh the initial utilization of ATP. Pumping sodium out of the cell and potassium into the cell has the added benefit of moving glucose into the cell at the same time.

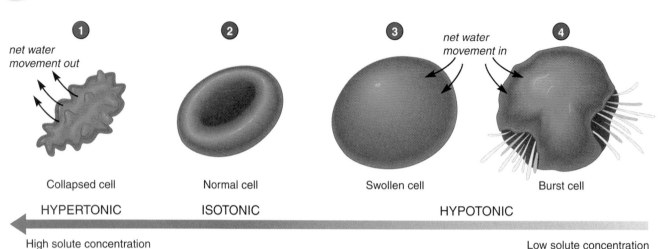

net water
movement out

net water
movement in

Collapsed cell   Normal cell   Swollen cell   Burst cell

HYPERTONIC   ISOTONIC   HYPOTONIC

High solute concentration
in extracellular fluid

Low solute concentration
in extracellular fluid

Figure 3-2 Tonicity.

Osmosis

Osmosis is the diffusion of water across a cell membrane. When molecules of solute are added to a solution, an equal number of molecules of solvent are displaced from the solution. For example, if 10 sodium ions are added to the fluid surrounding the cell, 10 molecules of water are displaced from that fluid. Therefore, the fluid surrounding the cell contains 10 fewer water molecules relative to the fluid within the cell. Water will diffuse down its concentration gradient to balance itself across the cell membrane. In this example, 5 water molecules will diffuse out of the cell into the surrounding fluid. Increasing the concentration of sodium in the surrounding (extracellular) fluid decreases the concentration of water in that fluid. Water diffuses out of the cell to create a balance of water molecules and to dilute the increased concentrations of sodium. Remember, where sodium goes, water follows.

The diffusion of water adds additional molecules to the extracellular compartment to create a balanced solution. This increased, yet balanced, volume puts pressure against the cell wall, called **osmotic pressure.** Osmotic pressure drives several important metabolic functions in the body, including cellular perfusion.

The effects of osmotic pressure on a cell are referred to as the **tonicity** of the solution (**Figure 3-2**). Tonicity is related to the concentration of sodium in a solution and the movement of water in relation to the sodium levels inside and outside the cell:

- An **isotonic solution** has the same concentration of sodium as does the cell. In this case, water doesn't shift, and no change in cell shape occurs.

- A **hypertonic solution** has a greater concentration of sodium than does the cell. Water is drawn out of the cell, and the cell collapses from the increased extracellular osmotic pressure.

- A **hypotonic solution** has a lower concentration of sodium than does the cell. Water flows into the cell, causing it to swell and possibly burst from the increased intracellular osmotic pressure.

IV fluids introduced into the circulatory system can affect the tonicity of the extracellular fluid, resulting in dire consequences unless care is used.

In osmosis, water diffuses across the cell membrane to reach a balance of equal concentration of water on either side of the cell membrane.

Fluid Compartments

The body stores water in various locations called fluid compartments. The fluid compartments are defined by their relationship to cells—the water is either inside the cell (intracellular) or outside the cell (extracellular). Although water levels in these compartments constantly shift, homeostatic control mechanisms ensure that balance is restored whenever water is lost.

The body's circulatory (vascular) system functions as a fluid highway, but it also contains cells. Thus, it can be thought of as another fluid compartment. Blood cells contain intracellular water and are surrounded by extracellular water. To differentiate between these two cellular areas, the extracellular compartment is broken down into:

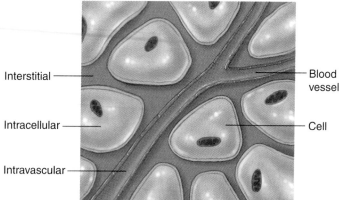

Figure 3-3 The three types of fluid compartments in the body.

- *Intravascular:* The water portion of the circulatory system surrounding the blood cells (for example in the heart, arteries, or veins)

- *Interstitial:* Water outside the vascular system and between surrounding cells (for example, between the membranes of two cells in muscle tissue)

In summary, there are three types of fluid compartments in the human body: intravascular (extracellular), interstitial (extracellular), and intracellular (**Figure 3-3**). The fluids within these compartments account for 60% of total body weight.

Intracellular fluid (ICF) accounts for 40% of total body weight, or two thirds of all fluid weight. ICF is within all the cells of the body. Large proteins within the cell can draw fluid into the cell because their overall negative charge attracts positively charged atoms like potassium, sodium, and the positive end of the water molecule (H_2O). The cell membrane prevents too many positively charged compounds, including water, from entering the cell and causing it to rupture. The sodium ions drawn into the cell are quickly removed via the **sodium/potassium pump** to prevent cellular **lysis.**

Extracellular fluid (ECF) occupies any area that is not inside the cells. Extracellular fluid compartments act as conduits for transferring gases and nutrients between the vascular and intracellular fluid compartments. ECF is found in the interstitial and intravascular compartments. ECF levels in the intravascular and interstitial compartments are regulated by the presence of sodium. Interstitial fluid accounts for 16% of total body weight and occupies the microscopic spaces between the cells. Interstitial fluid consists of a gel-type protein that helps disperse the water evenly throughout the interstitial compartment. This protein gel helps move water freely between the cells and vasculature. Intravascular fluid is also called plasma and accounts for 4% of total body weight. Perfusion occurs in the capillaries as a result of high hydrostatic pressures and osmosis in the **capillary beds.** The high arterial capillary pressures (hydrostatic pressures) placed on the capillary beds push fluids from the vascular compartment into the interstitial compartment.

sodium/potassium pump
The mechanism by which the cell brings in two potassium (K^+) ions and releases three sodium (Na^+) ions.

Dissolved oxygen and nutrients are carried along with the fluids. The resulting shift of fluids from the vascular system creates a high concentration of blood proteins in the venous side of the capillary, which pulls fluid back into the capillary circulation via osmosis.

Fluid Balance

Several factors influence the balance between ICF and ECF. The balance among intracellular, intravascular, and interstitial compartments is dynamic. Changes always occur, and the body adjusts to these changes by retaining or eliminating water. Fluid levels in the body are balanced when intakes equal outputs. Daily intakes of water include fluid from liquid, food, and cellular metabolism; daily outputs occur from respiration and excretion of urine and feces. **Table 3-1** demonstrates how fluid levels are controlled in the body. Amounts shown are estimates for fluid intake versus fluid output:

Table 3-1: Daily Fluid Balances

Fluid Gains	Daily Intake	Fluid Losses	Daily Output
Actual fluid intake	500-1,700 mL	Water vapor	850-1,200 mL
Fluid from solid food	800-1,000 mL	Urine	600-1,600 mL
Metabolism	200-300 mL	Feces	50-200 mL
Totals	1,500-3,000 mL	Totals	1,500-3,000 mL

The interstitial compartment is unique because it acts as the buffer between the other compartments. As fluid levels fluctuate between the intravascular and intracellular compartments, the interstitial compartment first responds by shifting **fluid reserves** between the two compartments (**Figure 3-4**). One clinical manifestation of a fluid imbalance is **edema**, which is defined as increased interstitial fluid levels. Causes of edema include:

- Increased arterial capillary pressures that push fluid out into the tissues (heart failure and/or unmonitored IV lines are possible causes)

- Decreased production of circulating blood proteins created in the liver, as seen with advanced liver diseases and severe burns

- Increased capillary permeability associated with capillary-dilating compounds, such as histamines released during allergic reactions

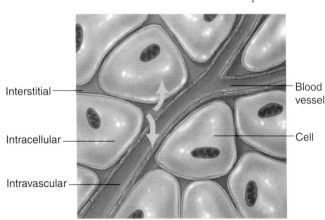

Interstitial — Blood vessel

Intracellular — Cell

Intravascular —

Figure 3-4 The interstitial compartment shifts fluid reserves.

Wrap Up

Chapter 3
Basic Cell Physiology

Ready for Review

In summary, the cellular environment contains ions, or electrolytes, that the cell uses for different purposes, depending on its needs. These ions include sodium (Na^+), potassium (K^+), calcium (Ca^+), bicarbonate (HCO_3^-), chloride (Cl^-), and phosphorus (Ph^{2-}). Their electrical charges must remain in balance on either side of the cell membrane. In addition, there must be a balance of compounds on either side of the cell membrane. If an imbalance occurs, the cell can move chemicals or charges across its membrane by various methods, including diffusion, filtration, active transport, and osmosis. Understanding the workings of extracellular and intracellular chemicals and charges will provide you with a better foundation for understanding why different types of IV fluids are administered for different conditions.

Quick Quiz

Answer each question below in your own words.

1 Define the term "electrolyte."

_____

_____

2 List the cellular cations.

_____

_____

3 List the cellular anions.

_____

_____

4 Explain why diffusion is kinetically favorable, whereas active transport is kinetically unfavorable.

_____

_____

5 Describe the process of osmosis.

_____

_____

_____

6 Explain tonicity and how it affects the cells of the body.

_____

_____

_____

7 List and compare the three types of fluid compartments found in the body.

_____

_____

_____

Principles of Fluid Balance

The role of water in the body is diverse; it plays a part both in **cellular metabolism** and in the maintenance of homeostasis. Without the presence of water in the body, people would quickly succumb to illness and disease, cellular function would cease, and body systems would shut down.

The role water plays in helping to maintain homeostasis is related to the size of the water molecule itself. Composed of only three atoms—two hydrogens and one oxygen—water has some unique properties (**Figure 4-1**). Water is a polar molecule—that is, it has a positive end (hydrogen) and a negative end (oxygen). This property means that water can surround charged particles and stabilize their charges, allowing the particles to remain in solution. Water can also move across cell membranes easily, because it is a relatively small molecule.

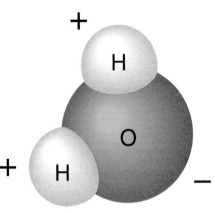

Figure 4-1 Water is a polar molecule with one positive end and one negative end.

Internal Environment of the Cell

The environment of the cells is one of water; some form of water surrounds all cells. Cells survive as long as this environment remains stable and is compatible for the life of the cell; any alteration in the supply of water, nutrients, oxygen, or food can lead to cellular death. Water exists both inside and outside the cell.

Homeostasis

Maintenance of the internal environment of the cell is regulated by elaborate systems of checks and balances. As systems in the body become imbalanced and begin to shift, feedback systems create an appropriate response to return the internal environment to normal. This normally balanced condition is referred to as **homeostasis**, or the resistance to change. These checks and balances can be seen in the way that the body regulates blood glucose: too little circulating blood glucose and the feedback system responds to create glucose; too much circulating blood glucose and the feedback system responds to store the excess glucose. When disturbances in homeostasis occur as a result of water shifting within the body, certain conditions develop related to the type of shifting that occurs.

Dehydration

Dehydration is defined as depletion of the body's total systemic fluid volume. Dehydration is usually a chronic condition of the elderly or the very young, and may take days to manifest. As fluid is lost from the vascular compartment, the body reacts by shifting interstitial fluid into the vascular area. This then forces a shift of fluid from the intracellular to the extracellular compartments. A total systemic fluid deficit occurs (**Figure 4-2**).

Signs and symptoms of dehydration include:

- Decreased **level of consciousness (LOC)**
- **Postural hypotension**
- **Tachypnea**
- Dry mucous membranes
- **Tachycardia**
- Poor skin turgor
- Flushed, dry skin

Causes of dehydration include:

- Diarrhea
- Vomiting
- Gastrointestinal (GI) drainage
- Hemorrhage
- Insufficient fluid/food intake

Overhydration

When the body's total systemic fluid volume increases, overhydration occurs. Fluid fills the vascular compartment, filters into the interstitial compartment, and finally is forced from the engorged interstitial compartment into the intracellular compartment. Fluid backup occurs, and the patient can succumb from these increased fluid levels (**Figure 4-3**).

Signs and symptoms of overhydration include:

- Shortness of breath
- Puffy eyelids
- Edema
- <u>Polyuria</u>
- Moist **crackles**
- Acute weight gain

Causes of overhydration include:

- Unmonitored IVs
- Kidney failure
- Prolonged **hypoventilation**

<u>homeostasis</u>
The body's resistance to change, here referring to the tendency of fluids located on either side of the cell wall to remain in balance.

<u>polyuria</u>
The passage of an unusually large volume of urine in a given period; in diabetes, polyuria can result from excreting excess glucose in the urine.

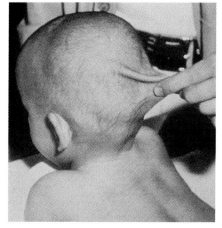

Figure 4-2 In a dehydrated patient, a total systemic deficit occurs.

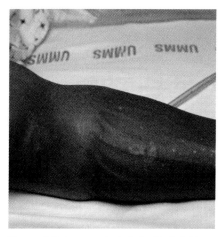

Figure 4-3 In an overhydrated patient, fluid backup occurs.

There are two ways to strengthen a solution: increase the amount of solute or decrease the amount of solvent.

Body Fluid Composition

The fluids found in the body are composed of dissolved elements and water, a combination known as a solution. A solution is a mixture of two things:

- *Solvent:* The fluid that does the dissolving, or the solution that contains the dissolved components (in the body, the solvent is water)

- *Solute:* The dissolved particles contained in the solvent

A good example of making a solution is the process of brewing a cup of coffee. Passing hot water (solvent) over the ground beans leaches out the oils (the solute) to create the solution know as coffee. Remember, as the solute concentration increases, the solvent concentration decreases. Is a strong cup of coffee created by using less water (solvent) or by adding more coffee (solute)? Either one could be true, as they both end up creating stronger coffee.

Acid/Base Balance

Homeostasis requires a balance between acids and bases in the body. An **acid** can be defined as any molecule that gives up a hydrogen ion and is often referred to as H^+. A **base** is defined as any molecule that can accept a hydrogen ion and is often referred to as OH^-. Acids can be further classified as either strong or weak, depending on how completely they **disassociate** in water. Strong acids like hydrogen chloride (HCl) disassociate almost completely, whereas weak acids like carbonic acid (H_2CO_3) only partially disassociate. It is the ability of weak acids to bond weakly to hydrogen ions that makes them ideal buffers, as they can either accept or donate hydrogen ions, depending on the needs of the body. Several mechanisms help regulate the acids and bases created during normal metabolism.

Defining the Acidity of a Solution

pH
A measure of the acidity of a solution.

The acidity of a solution is defined by the amount of free hydrogen found in the solution. The measurement of hydrogen in solution is called **pH**. Measurement of pH is based on the ratio of the amount of acid (H^+) to the amount of base (OH^-). One H^+ removes one OH^- from solution, creating H_2O, so if there is exactly enough H^+ for every OH^-, the result is pure water (neither acidic nor basic) with a pH of 7. Thus, the definition of neutral pH is based on the equation:

$$[H^+] \ + \ [OH^-] \ \leftrightarrow \ [H_2O]$$

If there are more H^+ ions in solution than OH^-, the solution becomes acidic (pH below 7), and the pH drops. If there are fewer H^+ ions in solution than OH^-, the solution becomes basic (pH above 7), and the pH rises. Normal body functions work best within the very narrow pH between 7.35 and 7.45. Cellular function deteriorates and death occurs when the pH drops below 6.9 or rises above 7.8.

It is important to note that concentrations of H^+ ions can be increased either by adding more H^+ ions *or* by removing OH^-. To illustrate this concept, remember the coffee example. To make strong coffee, you can either add more coffee grounds or you can add less water. The reverse is also true to make the solution basic.

Ion Shifts

In order to function properly, an acid/base balance, or balance of charges, must exist on either side of the cell. If excess hydrogen ions exist in the extracellular fluid around a cell, diffusion occurs, and hydrogen ions move into the cell along the charge gradient between the extracellular and intracellular fluids. When hydrogen moves across the cell membrane into the cell, the cell starts taking on an overall positive charge. To return its overall charge to neutral, the cell begins to shift cations into the interstitial fluid. Hydrogen ions moving into the cell force potassium to shift out into the extracellular fluid until no more potassium can safely be shifted out of the cell. This shift has significant consequences. Decreasing intracellular potassium leads to problems with cellular depolarization. High serum (intravascular) potassium levels (hyperkalemia) mean the cell needs a greater stimulus to depolarize.

Calcium (Ca^{2+}) ions also shift out of the cell in response to the influx of hydrogen. **Neural permeability** is regulated by the presence calcium ions. High serum calcium levels (hypercalcemia) decrease **neural transmissions,** whereas low serum calcium levels (hypocalcemia) lead to hypersensitive nerve cells and increased neural transmissions. In summary, an increase in extracellular hydrogen ions results in acidosis; a decrease in extracellular hydrogen ions results in alkalosis.

> ↑pH means ↓H^+ ion concentration = alkalosis
> ↓pH means ↑H^+ ion concentration = acidosis

Buffers

A buffer is a compound that can repeatedly neutralize excess acids or bases to prevent pH levels from exceeding acceptable levels. Several different buffers and buffering sites exist in the body:

- Circulating proteins can bind with excess acids or bases, thus neutralizing their effects.

- Bone acts as a buffer by absorbing excess acids and bases and by releasing calcium into circulation.

- The bicarbonate buffer system circulates in all fluid compartments of the body.

When buffers become dysfunctional, the patient is more likely to develop acidosis or alkalosis and thus more likely to need IV therapy.

Any buffer system in the body may be best imagined as a bucket. Like a bucket, the buffer system can only hold a certain amount of acid before it reaches the point where it is saturated and overflows. The body responds to shifts in pH levels by either absorbing or releasing small amounts of acid into the blood. Problems begin when the amount of acid in circulation is too great and the buffer system becomes overwhelmed.

There are three main components to the buffer system found in the body:

- The circulating bicarbonate buffer component
- The respiratory component
- The renal component

The following equation illustrates the balance among these three components:

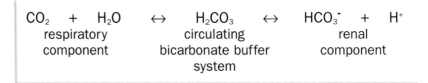

$$CO_2 \;+\; H_2O \quad\leftrightarrow\quad H_2CO_3 \quad\leftrightarrow\quad HCO_3^- \;+\; H^+$$

respiratory component · circulating bicarbonate buffer system · renal component

The Circulating Bicarbonate Buffer Component

This component is the "bucket" that holds and neutralizes excess acid. The circulating bicarbonate buffer system can be found in the intracellular and extracellular fluids and is the fastest acting segment of the buffer system.

$$H_2CO_3 \quad\leftrightarrow\quad H^+ \;+\; HCO_3^-$$

Carbonic acid (H_2CO_3) is a weak acid that can give up an extra hydrogen ion (H^+) to reform as the bicarbonate ion (HCO_3^-). Through metabolic processes, the extra H^+ is then converted into compounds that are easily expelled from the body, eliminating the extra acid.

The Respiratory Component

$$H_2CO_3 \quad\leftrightarrow\quad CO_2 \;+\; H_2O$$

The fastest way the body can get rid of the excess H^+ ions is to create water (H_2O) and carbon dioxide (CO_2), which can be expelled as gases in the lungs. The preceding equation illustrates this process, which occurs in the lungs.

The main reason for breathing is to maintain the circulating level of carbon dioxide in the blood. Carbon dioxide combines with the circulating water of the blood to create carbonic acid (H_2CO_3). Chemoreceptors in the brain sense the rising levels of carbonic acid and signal the respiratory center to increase ventilation and to reduce the available amount of circulating carbon dioxide. Tachypnea then reduces the level of carbon

If a patient's respiratory rate is too low, acidosis is likely to develop. If a patient's respiratory rate is too high, alkalosis is likely to develop.

dioxide. Although the respiratory component reacts within minutes, it is much slower to respond than the circulating buffer system. Using the buffer bucket example, the respiratory component can be thought of as a large faucet that allows acid to spill out of the buffer bucket, returning the pH to normal levels.

$$\text{Excess } H^+ \Rightarrow H_2CO_3 \Rightarrow CO_2 \Rightarrow \text{Tachypnea}$$

Anything that limits respirations can lead to acid retention and acidosis. Any time a patient is in respiratory distress or is unable to breathe, acidosis quickly develops.

$$\text{Bradypnea} \Rightarrow \uparrow CO_2 \Rightarrow \uparrow H_2CO_3 \Rightarrow \text{acidosis}$$

The preceding equation demonstrates how a patient experiencing respiratory difficulty drives the respiratory component back toward acid retention. The patient can also experience alkalosis if the respiratory rate is too high, as shown in the equation below.

$$\text{Tachypnea} \Rightarrow \downarrow CO_2 \Rightarrow \downarrow H_2CO_3 \Rightarrow \text{alkalosis}$$

The Renal Component

$$H_2CO_3 \leftrightarrow H^+ + HCO_3^-$$

Another smaller faucet connected to the buffer bucket is the renal component. The smaller faucet size represents the slower nature by which the kidneys respond to increasing acid levels. The renal response could take from hours to days to restore the body's pH to normal. Kidneys account for every molecule, ion, and electrolyte found in the circulation.

As with the respiratory system, the renal system can control increasing acid levels in the blood by excreting the acid. The kidneys excrete acid in an ionic form, unlike the respiratory system, which excretes acid as a gas.

> If a patient cannot urinate, acidosis is likely to develop. If a patient urinates excessively, alkalosis is likely to develop.

$$\text{Excess } H^+ \Rightarrow H_2CO_3 \Rightarrow HCO_3^- + H^+ \text{(urine)}$$

If the patient experiences decreased urine output, excess acid cannot be removed from the blood, and the patient can experience acidosis.

$$\text{Decreased output} \Rightarrow \uparrow H^+ \Rightarrow \uparrow HCO_3^- \Rightarrow \text{acidosis}$$

If urine output becomes excessive, alkalosis can develop.

$$\text{Increased output} \Rightarrow \downarrow H^+ \Rightarrow \downarrow HCO_3^- \Rightarrow \text{alkalosis}$$

Compensatory Mechanisms

Acid/base disorders that are not immediately correctable by the body's buffering systems cause compensatory mechanisms to begin in order to help return levels to normal. A **metabolic acidosis** may create a **respiratory alkalosis** as a compensatory response. Often, patient management involves treating more than one form of acid/base imbalance.

Clinical Presentations

There are two types of acid/base disorders: metabolic and respiratory.

- Fluctuations in pH due to available bicarbonate levels result in metabolic acidosis or alkalosis.
- Fluctuations in pH due to respiratory disorders result in respiratory acidosis or alkalosis.

This results in four main clinical presentation combinations:

- Respiratory acidosis
- Metabolic acidosis
- Respiratory alkalosis
- Metabolic alkalosis

Respiratory Acidosis

$$\downarrow \text{Breathing} \Rightarrow \uparrow CO_2 \Rightarrow \uparrow H_2CO_3 \Rightarrow \downarrow pH$$

Respiratory acidosis is always related to hypoventilation of some type. Because, the acidosis problem is a result of insufficient breathing, the compensatory mechanism is the slower reacting renal system. Some causes for respiratory acidosis are:

- Airway obstruction
- Cardiac arrest
- Narcotic drug use
- Drowning
- Respiratory arrest
- **Pulmonary edema**
- Closed head injury
- Chest trauma
- Carbon monoxide (CO) poisoning

> **R**espiratory acidosis and alkalosis are caused by ventilation problems. Acidosis and alkalosis that result from any other cause are called metabolic.

Hypoventilation that develops from any of the conditions listed above is considered a serious, life-threatening condition. The acidosis that results is quick, overwhelming, and usually fatal, making it impossible for the slower-reacting renal system to compensate in time for the pH shift. The increasing acidosis causes potassium ions to shift into the extracellular fluid, leading to fatal **cardiac dysrhythmias.** Calcium also shifts into extracellular spaces, resulting in hypercalcemia and decreased neural cell permeability and creating lethargy and a decreasing LOC.

Signs and symptoms of respiratory acidosis include:

- Systemic/**cerebral vasodilation**
- Headaches
- Red, flushed skin
- **Central nervous system (CNS) depression**
- **Bradypnea**
- Nausea and vomiting
- Hypercalcemia

These signs and symptoms help explain why patients with **diabetic ketoacidosis (DKA)** may have red, flushed skin and patients with carbon monoxide poisoning may have severe headaches.

When assessing patients for respiratory acidosis, evaluate:

- LOC
- Skin color and temperature
- Respiratory rate and effort
- Lung sounds
- Hydration
- Cardiac rhythm changes

diabetic ketoacidosis (DKA)
A form of acidosis in uncontrolled diabetes in which an accumulation of certain acids occurs when insulin is not available in the body.

A Brief Word About COPD

Chronic obstructive pulmonary disease (COPD) creates respiratory acidosis over time. It is that slow onset that makes this form of respiratory acidosis survivable as compared to other forms of respiratory acidosis. The gradual destruction of lung tissue inhibits the exchange of oxygen and carbon dioxide, creating acidosis. With COPD, the normal stimulus for this exchange is absent. Increasing carbon dioxide retention leads to increasing levels of carbonic acid, eventually making chemoreceptors unaware of the presence of metabolic acids. **Hypoxic drive** is then the only stimulus for respiration left. Hypoxic drive relies on circulating oxygen levels as its marker. The chronic nature of COPD allows the renal system enough time to moderate the acidosis, thus preventing the life-threatening cardiac dysrhythmias that occur from acute acidosis.

Healthy individuals also respond to oxygen and carbon dioxide levels in the blood. When oxygen levels rise too high, the respiratory center suspends respiration until rising carbon dioxide levels stimulate the respiratory center to begin breathing again. With COPD, the rising carbon dioxide levels never stimulate the respiratory center to begin breathing again. This presents a dilemma: COPD patients in respiratory distress need ventilatory assistance with high-flow oxygen even though it may suppress their respiratory drive and create respiratory arrest. Respiratory arrest, though, can be treated.

Respiratory Alkalosis

$$\uparrow Breathing \implies \downarrow CO_2 \implies \downarrow H_2CO_3 \implies \uparrow pH$$

Respiratory alkalosis is always the result of **hyperventilation.** Carbon dioxide levels drop in the blood, forcing a reduction of circulating carbonic acid. The renal system then begins retaining hydrogen ions to rebalance the depleted acid levels. As this is happening, hydrogen ions begin to shift from the extracellular to the intracellular fluid compartments. Calcium shifts into the intracellular compartment to rebalance depleted hydrogen levels. Hypocalcemia leads to increased neural cell permeability. Muscle contractions create the classic signs of carpal/pedal spasms that accompany hyperventilation. Treatment for the classic hyperventilation syndrome focuses on restoring the normal respiratory rate to increase carbon dioxide levels. However, increasing carbon dioxide levels can aggravate other more serious medical conditions that produce hyperventilation. That is why you must evaluate the reason for the hyperventilation before you attempt to correct it.

Some effects of respiratory alkalosis include:

- Decreased **cerebral perfusion**
- Vertigo
- Decreased LOC
- Blurred vision
- Lightheadedness
- Hypocalcemia
- Confusion
- Nausea and vomiting

When assessing these patients, evaluate:

- LOC
- Lung sounds
- Skin color and temperature
- Hydration
- Respiratory rate and effort
- Cardiac rhythm changes

Some causes for hyperventilation and respiratory alkalosis can be:

- Drug overdoses, especially aspirin
- Improper bag-valve-mask (BVM) technique
- Fever

Metabolic Acidosis

$$\uparrow H_2CO_3 \Rightarrow \uparrow H^+ + HCO_3^- \Rightarrow \downarrow pH$$

Any acidosis that is not related to the respiratory system is considered metabolic in origin. Tachypnea is the compensatory mechanism for these patients as the respiratory system attempts to restore acid/base balance by eliminating carbon dioxide. Patient presentations for metabolic acidosis are similar to those for respiratory acidosis.

As with any acidosis, extracellular hydrogen levels increase, and the extracellular buffers attempt to neutralize the excess acid. Ion shifts occur, hydrogen leaks into the cell, and potassium shifts into the extracellular spaces, raising the serum potassium levels, which can lead to potentially life-threatening cardiac dysrhythmias. Along with the potassium ion shift, calcium also shifts into extracellular spaces. The resulting hypercalcemia leads to decreased neural cell permeability. Impulses sent to muscle and nerve cells are obstructed, and the patient becomes lethargic with a decreased LOC.

Major causes for metabolic acidosis include:

- **Lactic acidosis** created by anaerobic cellular respiration due to **hypoperfusion** of tissues and organs, as seen with shock and cardiac arrest.

- **Ketoacidosis** resulting when cells are forced to switch to metabolizing fatty acids for energy because they are unable to utilize glucose, either because of insulin insufficiency or desensitization of the cells to insulin. The by-products of fat metabolism are **ketones,** which are extremely acidotic.

- Aspirin (acetylsalicylic acid) overdose (10 to 30 g for adults). Acetylsalicylic acid directly stimulates the respiratory centers of the brain, creating tachypnea and leading to respiratory alkalosis. Compensatory mechanisms involve the renal system, resulting in metabolic acidosis.

- Alcohol ingestion. Ingestion of ethyl alcohol can lead to **alcoholic ketoacidosis.** Methanol (wood alcohol) and ethylene glycol can produce fatal forms of acidosis, often with amounts as small as 30 mL.

- GI losses. Diarrhea, for example, removes bases from the lower intestinal tract.

Signs and symptoms of metabolic acidosis include:

- Vasodilation
- CNS depression
- Headaches
- Hot, red, flushed skin
- Hypercalcemia
- Tachypnea
- Nausea and vomiting
- Dysrhythmias

When assessing patients with metabolic acidosis, evaluate:

- LOC
- Skin color and temperature
- Respiratory effort and rate
- Lung sounds
- Hydration
- Cardiac rhythm

Metabolic Alkalosis

$$\downarrow H^+ \Rightarrow \downarrow H_2CO_3^- \Rightarrow \uparrow pH \Rightarrow \text{bradypnea}$$

Metabolic alkalosis results anytime there is excessive loss of acid, either from excessive urination or from decreased acid levels in the stomach. Several factors related to upper GI losses can lead to metabolic alkalosis:

- Excessive vomiting
- Excessive water intake
- Nasogastric suctioning
- Excessive intake of base
- Eating disorders

Major causes for metabolic alkalosis are as follows:

- Upper GI losses of acid resulting from illness or anorexia. When the patient expels a great deal of acid from the stomach, a complex metabolic pathway can lead to metabolic alkalosis.

- Drinking large amounts of water during heavy exertion. The water not only dilutes the stomach acid, it also stimulates the digestive system to prepare for incoming food from the stomach. This stimulation causes a dump of very basic digestive enzymes into the lower GI tract, adding to the acid/base imbalance. As with respiratory alkalosis, there is a shift of calcium out of the cell—hypercalcemia—causing overstimulation of the nervous system and leading to muscle cramping. This cramping is analogous to carpal/pedal spasms, except it occurs in the abdominal area and is referred to as **heat cramps.**

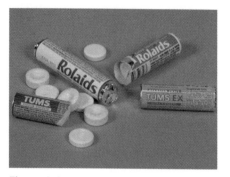

Figure 4-4 Excessive intake of base-like antacids can result in metabolic alkalosis.

- Excessive intake of base-like antacids (**Figure 4-4**). This is important to remember when dealing with cardiac patients, because one of their main complaints tends to be feelings of nausea or indigestion. Often, the patient has self-medicated for hours or days with over-the-counter antacids, which can result in metabolic alkalosis. Another cause of excessive base intake is the use of sodium bicarbonate ($NaHCO_3$) through an IV line. Introducing one ampoule (amp) of sodium bicarbonate through an IV line can seriously alter pH levels.

The compensatory mechanism for metabolic alkalosis is the respiratory system. To correct the reduced hydrogen levels, bradypnea develops to retain carbon dioxide and drive up the levels of circulating acids.

Signs and symptoms of metabolic alkalosis include:

- Confusion
- Muscle tremors and cramps
- Bradypnea
- Hypotension

IV Fluid Composition

IV solutions are tools designed to facilitate patient treatment. The use of IV fluids can significantly alter the patient's condition. It is critical that each bag of IV solution be sterile and safe; therefore, each bag of IV solution is individually sterilized (**Figure 4-5**). Compounds and ions dissolved in the solution are identical to the ones found in the body. Each solution is a concentration of solute and solvent.

Because sodium is the primary extracellular cation and regulates water levels in the body, it is used as the benchmark to calculate a solution's tonicity. The concentration of sodium in the cells of the body is 0.9%. Altering the concentration of sodium in the IV solution can move the water into or out of any fluid compartment in the body. Remember, where sodium goes, water follows.

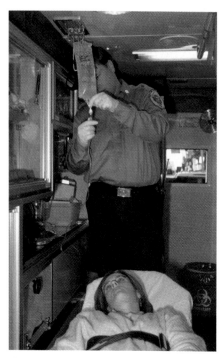

Figure 4-5 It is imperative that each bag of IV solution be sterile and safe.

Types of IV Solutions

There are five basic types of IV solutions, each with a different tonicity and dissolved components. The five basic types are isotonic, hypotonic, hypertonic, crystalloid, and colloid. IV fluids use combinations of these five types of solutions to create the desired effects inside the body.

Isotonic Solutions

Isotonic solutions possess close to the same **osmolarity** as serum and other body fluids. Because there is no alteration of serum osmolarity, the fluid stays inside the intravascular compartment. Isotonic solutions

> IV fluids have many of the same components as body fluids.
>
> Therefore, fluid insufficiencies in the body can be corrected through IV therapy.

expand the contents of the intravascular compartment without shifting fluid to or from other compartments. Awareness of this fact is useful when dealing with hypotensive or hypovolemic patients. Because this fluid remains in the vascular compartment, you must be careful to avoid fluid overloading. Patients with **hypertension** and **congestive heart failure** are at greatest risk of fluid overload. The extra fluid increases the workload of the heart, creating fluid backup in the lungs. **Lactated Ringer's (LR)** solution isn't normally used in the field because it contains the buffering compound lactate. LR solution should not be given to patients with liver problems because they cannot metabolize the lactate.

D_5W—5% dextrose in water—is a special type of isotonic solution. As long as it remains in the bag, it is considered an isotonic solution. Once it is administered, the dextrose is quickly metabolized, and the solution becomes hypotonic.

Hypotonic Solutions

A hypotonic fluid has an osmolarity less than that of serum—that is, it has less sodium ion concentration than serum. When this fluid is placed in the vascular compartment, it begins diluting the serum. Soon the serum osmolarity is less than the interstitial fluid; water is pulled from the vascular compartment into the interstitial fluid compartment and eventually the same process is repeated, pulling water from the interstitial compartment into the cells.

Hypotonic solutions hydrate the cells while depleting the vascular compartment. These solutions may be needed for a patient on dialysis when diuretic therapy dehydrates the cells. They may also be used for hyperglycemic conditions like diabetic ketoacidosis, in which high serum glucose levels draw fluid out of the cells and into the vascular and interstitial compartments. Hypotonic solutions can be dangerous to use because they can cause a sudden fluid shift from the intravascular space to the cells, causing cardiovascular collapse and increased **intracranial pressure (ICP)** from shifting fluid into the brain cells. For example, giving D_5W for an extended period can cause increased ICP. This makes hypotonic solutions dangerous to use with patients experiencing a **stroke** or any head trauma. Using hypotonic solutions on patients with burns, trauma, malnutrition, or liver disease is also hazardous, because these patients are at risk for developing **third spacing,** an abnormal fluid shift into the **serous linings** of the body.

Hypertonic Solutions

A hypertonic solution has an osmolarity higher than serum—that is, it has more **ionic concentration** than serum and pulls fluid and electrolytes from the intracellular and interstitial compartments into the intravascular compartment. Hypertonic solutions shift body fluids into the vascular spaces and help stabilize blood pressure, increase urine output, and reduce edema. These fluids are rarely, if ever, used in the prehospital setting. Often, the term "hypertonic" refers to solutions that contain high concentrations of proteins because they have the same effect on fluid as sodium. Careful monitoring is needed to guard against fluid overloading when using hypertonic fluids, especially with patients who suffer from impaired heart or kidney function. Also, hypertonic solutions

An example of a hypotonic solution is D5NS.45– 5% dextrose in ½ normal saline.

Examples of hypertonic solutions are 9.0% NS, blood products, and albumin.

Albumin and steroids are examples of colloid solutions.

should not be given to patients with diabetic ketoacidosis or others at risk of cellular dehydration. Hypertonic solutions have been studied in the treatment of patients experiencing hemorrhaging to help restore blood pressure while minimizing fluid overloading.

Crystalloid Solutions

Crystalloid solutions contain compounds that quickly disassociate in solution. The ability of these fluids to cross membranes and alter the various fluid levels makes them the best choice for the prehospital care of injured patients who need fluid replacement for body fluid loss. When using an isotonic crystalloid for fluid replacement to support blood pressure from blood loss, remember the 3 to 1 replacement rule: *3 mL of isotonic crystalloid solution are needed to replace 1 mL of patient blood.* This is because approximately two thirds of the infused crystalloid solution will leave the vascular spaces in about 1 hour.

Colloid Solutions

Colloid solutions contain molecules (usually proteins) that are too large to pass out of the capillary membranes and therefore remain in the vascular compartment. The very large protein molecules give colloid solutions a very high osmolarity. As a result, they draw fluid from the interstitial and intracellular compartments into the vascular compartments. Colloid solutions work very well in reducing edema (as in **pulmonary** or **cerebral edema**) while expanding the vascular compartment. These fluids could cause dramatic fluid shifts and place the patient in considerable danger if they are not administered in a controlled setting. Examples of colloids are albumin and steroids.

Blood

There are 5 million red blood cells, 7,500 white blood cells, and 3 million platelet cells in 1 cubic millimeter of blood, making up the **formed elements** of blood. The sticky liquid portion of the blood (called the plasma) constitutes the **nonformed elements** of the blood. It is interesting to note that red blood cells live only about 120 days and are replaced in the body at a rate of a few million red blood cells per second.

Nonformed Elements

Nonformed elements account for approximately 55% of total blood volume. Plasma is the main component of the nonformed elements and is responsible for moving all the other formed elements of the blood. Plasma is approximately 90% water and carries the following:

- All of the nutrients needed by the cells to stay alive

- Waste products of the cells

- Antibodies

Formed Elements

Formed elements account for 45% of the total blood volume. **Erythrocytes,** or red blood cells (RBCs), are the primary formed element and are unique. They contain ferrous (iron) rings called **heme rings.** Heme rings have the ability to bind with oxygen to form **oxyhemoglobin** (**Figure 4-6**). Oxyhemoglobin delivers oxygen to the cells of the body. At the cellular level, the bound oxygen is shifted off the heme ring and transported out of the vascular compartment and into the interstitial compartment.

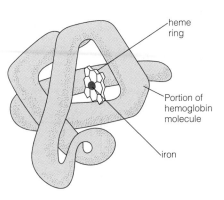

Figure 4-6 The heme ring of the hemoglobin molecule has the ability to bind to oxygen.

A Brief Discussion of Cyanosis

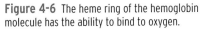

People who cannot make enough red blood cells may develop **iron deficiency anemia** because they lack enough iron to create heme rings. Less hemoglobin production means less oxygen transported to cells, which leads to decreased cellular function. Normal human blood contains 15 g of hemoglobin per 100 mL of blood. Anemic patients often have less than that, often as low as 6 g/100 mL of blood. These low levels of hemoglobin translate to less oxygen-carrying capabilities in anemic patients.

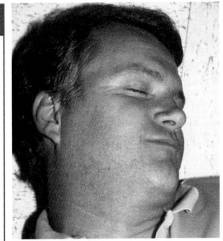

Figure 4-7. A patient presenting with cyanosis.

Often, cyanosis is used as a sign of **hypoxia** (**Figure 4-7**). However, relying on cyanosis can present a problem, particularly in a patient with anemia. The bluish tinge associated with cyanosis appears in patients when more than 5 g of hemoglobin becomes desaturated in normal blood circulation. Truly anemic patients could have as little as 6 g of hemoglobin per 100 mL (less than half the normal level of hemoglobin). Patients with anemia can have as much as 3 g of hemoglobin desaturated per 100 mL of blood and will not show any signs of cyanosis even though 50% of their blood is desaturated. A pulse oximetry reading for these patients could be as low as 50%.

Thrombocytes (Platelets)

Platelets plug holes in damaged vessels of the circulatory system through a long and involved activation process that requires numerous blood components. Basically, platelets flow through the extremely smooth vessel linings until they encounter a rough area of vessel damage, which causes them to rupture. **Clotting factors** are released, causing more platelets to aggregate at the site, rupture, and repeat the cycle until the damage is controlled. The rupturing platelets trigger **prothrombin** to form **thrombin.** In the last step, thrombin combines with **fibrinogen** to form a water-insoluble gel called **fibrin.** This is the hard scab that covers wounds. Blood clots can also form internally in the vessels, sometimes leading to blockages in arteries that can cause tissue death. If the blockage occurs in the coronary arteries, an **infarct** exists.

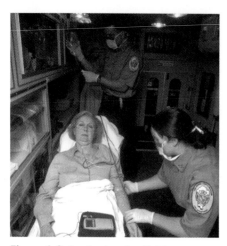

Figure 4-8 New treatments with intravenous drugs can assist in dissolving clots.

New treatments for clots involve activating the body's own clot-dissolving mechanisms with drugs introduced into the circulation intravenously (**Figure 4-8**). This is an important concept to remember when treating a stationary clot (thrombus) in the vascular circulation of the heart and brain. Some of the more common drugs in use are streptokinase and tPA. For these drugs to work, they must be administered within a narrow window of time. It is very important not to waste IV sites when treating patients who have experienced cardiac arrest or **cerebrovascular accidents (CVAs)**, because multiple IV sites will be needed at the hospital, and unsuccessful sites will bleed when these drugs are used.

Blood Types

Blood cells can be identified by their **surface antigens** (an antigen stimulates an immune response). These surface antigens act like name tags. **Macrophages** and antibodies check the name tags to be sure the blood belongs in circulation. If a cell does not have the proper identification, it is destroyed. There are four blood group types. Every person fits into one of these four blood types, listed in **Table 4-1**:

Table 4-1 Blood Type Groupings		
Blood Type	**Surface Antigen**	**Circulating Antibodies**
A	A	B
B	B	A
AB	AB	None – universal recipient
O	None – universal donor	AB

The letter stands for the antigen present on the surface of the blood cell and indicates there are no circulating antibodies targeting that specific surface antigen. So, for example, if you have type A blood, you have anti-B antibodies and no anti-A antibodies. If you are type AB, your serum contains neither anti-A or anti-B antibodies. If you are type O, your blood cells contain no surface antigens to elicit an immune response. Universal donors are blood type O and universal recipients are type AB. Introduction of an incompatible blood type can cause a serious transfusion reaction. The entire infused amount of blood can clump and clog all circulation in the area.

Rh Factor

The **Rh factor** was discovered during experiments conducted on rhesus monkeys during research in blood chemistry. If someone has the additional Rh surface antigen, they are said to be Rh⁺. The Rh factor is relatively insignificant except in the case of an Rh⁻ woman pregnant by an Rh⁺ man. The Rh⁺ factor is the dominant genetic trait and will most likely produce an Rh⁺ child. When the child is born, and if maternal blood is exposed to fetal blood, the mother will begin antibody production targeted toward the Rh⁺ fetal blood. During the next pregnancy (assuming that the father is again Rh⁺), the Rh⁺ fetus and the Rh⁻ mother are both at high risk for immune system attacks on the foreign blood protein. This reaction can be life threatening for both mother and child. Fortunately, there is a way to prevent this reaction. If an Rh⁻ mother gives birth to an Rh⁺ baby, the mother is given a single dose of RhoGAM, an immune globulin designed to prevent the development of anti-Rh⁺ antibodies. Mothers receive this shot after every birth to prevent fatal reactions in future pregnancies (**Figure 4-9**).

Fluid Measurements

Often, you will hear emergency department (ED) staff talk about the "crit" levels of patients brought into the ED. A **hematocrit** is a common laboratory test to measure the amounts of formed and unformed elements of the blood. In this test, a test tube of blood is placed in a **centrifuge** at 10,000 rpm to separate the sample into red blood cells, white blood cells, and plasma by density. The test is designed to measure the percentage of blood components circulating in a patient's vasculature. A normal sample has a red blood cell count of 35% to 45%—that is, a crit value between 35 and 45. **Figure 4-10** shows a hematocrit test that exhibits ideal blood component values.

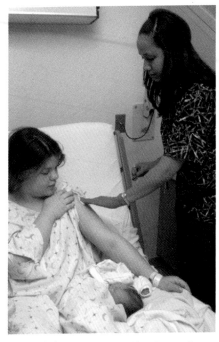

Figure 4-9 RhoGAM can be given to a mother after birth to prevent the development of anti Rh+ antibodies.

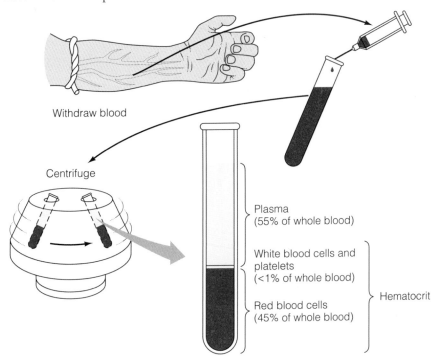

Figure 4-10 Hemocrit test.

Withdraw blood

Centrifuge

Plasma (55% of whole blood)

White blood cells and platelets (<1% of whole blood)

Red blood cells (45% of whole blood)

Hematocrit

Blood Transfusion Complications

Transfusion reactions are rare, but it is important to recognize one developing if you are assisting in the ED with a patient receiving blood. Some of the more common transfusion reactions produce only a slight temperature, whereas others produce life-threatening reactions. Common reactions include the following:

- Fever, which can be caused from sensitivity of the recipient's immune system to the foreign proteins in the donor's blood.

- Allergic reactions, such as **urticaria**.

- Clinical signs and symptoms of viral hepatitis.

- Hemolytic reactions, which can arise from as little as 50 mL of donor blood.

- Acute, sharp lower back pain caused by the kidneys getting clogged from the clumping blood; chest pain; acute, worsening shortness of breath resulting from the decreasing availability of circulating blood cells needed for the exchange of oxygen and carbon dioxide; and/or severe headache related to the developing acidosis. A conscious patient may complain of these symptoms. However, an unconscious patient cannot verbalize complaints. The unconscious patient may show:

  - Flushed skin followed by cyanosis

  - Cool and clammy skin with **diaphoresis**

  - Bradycardia

  - **Jugular vein distention (JVD)**

  - Drop in blood pressure

If you suspect any type of transfusion reaction, you need to take the following steps:

1. Stop the transfusion *immediately* (see "Discontinuing the IV Line" in Chapter 7, page 86).

2. Start an additional line of normal saline.

3. Draw a blood sample from the arm opposite the infusion to avoid obtaining a sample with transfusion-initiated clotting.

4. Contact medical control immediately.

urticaria
Small spots of generalized itching and/or burning that appear as multiple raised areas on the skin; hives.

Wrap Up

Chapter 4
Principles of Fluid Balance

Ready for Review

Proper pH balance is crucial for the body to function properly. An acid/base imbalance can lead to alkalosis or acidosis, both of which require medical intervention. IV therapy can be used to correct these problems. You can prepare yourself for these situations by learning the signs and symptoms of respiratory and metabolic acidosis and alkalosis. Finally, becoming familiar with the five types of IV solutions will give you an understanding of their use in relation to patient conditions.

Quick Quiz

Answer each question below in your own words.

1. Explain the acid/base concept in terms of pH.
   _____

2. Explain the differences between the four acid/base clinical patient presentations.
   _____

3. Explain the differences between the five types of IV solutions.
   _____

4. Explain the differences between all the formed and nonformed elements of blood.
   _____

5. Briefly explain the concept of ion shifting.
   _____

6. Why is a weak acid considered a buffer?
   _____

7. Explain the correlation between acids and bases and the pH scale.
   _____

8. Fill in the blanks with the appropriate numbers, words, or symbols:
   a. Acidosis = _____ in pH.
   b. Alkalosis = _____ in pH.
   c. Bradypnea $\Rightarrow$ _____ CO_2 $\Rightarrow$ _____ H_2CO_3 $\Rightarrow$ _____
   d. Tachypnea $\Rightarrow$ _____ CO_2 $\Rightarrow$ _____ H_2CO_3 $\Rightarrow$ _____
   e. $\uparrow$ Extracellular H^+ $\Rightarrow$ _____ of intracellular H^+, which leads to a shift of intracellular _____ out of the cell, which leads to _____ of serum electrolytes.
   f. $\downarrow$ Extracellular H^+ $\Rightarrow$ _____ of intracellular H^+, which leads to a shift of intracellular _____ out of the cell, which leads to _____ of serum electrolytes.
   g. An acid has pH below _____.
   h. A base has pH above _____.
   i. Respiratory _____ always results from tachypnea.
   j. Respiratory _____ always results from bradypnea.

Causes and Treatment of Shock

Of all the possible injuries or illnesses you will encounter, none is as serious or as easy to prevent as shock. **Shock** is defined as inadequate tissue oxygenation and **perfusion**. The treatment of shock is a **basic life support (BLS)** skill that EMTs of all certification levels must know. It is therefore important to recognize its presence.

Causes of Shock

The human circulatory system can be thought of as a closed hydraulic system made up of a pump, hoses, and fluid (**Figure 5-1**). This system produces pressure to keep tissues oxygenated. Failure of any one of the components can lead to shock. Failure of the pump (the heart) results in inadequate pressure, leading to cardiogenic or obstructive shock. Types of hose (vessel) failure include vasogenic, neurogenic, septic, and anaphylactic shock. Finally, failure of the circulating fluid to provide enough volume for tissue **perfusion** results in fluid shock, which includes **hypovolemia, hemorrhagic shock,** and third spacing shock.

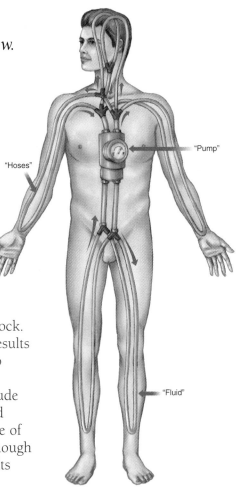

"Pump"

"Hoses"

"Fluid"

Figure 5-1 The human circulatory system is a closed hydraulic system.

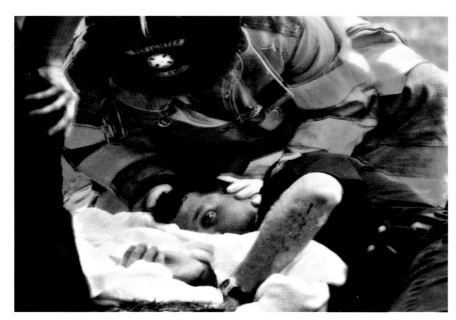

Figure 5-2 A patient in shock.

<u>perfusion</u>
The circulation of blood within an organ or tissue in adequate amounts to meet the cell's current needs.

<u>hypoxia</u>
A dangerous condition in which the body tissues and cells do not have enough oxygen.

Tissue perfusion depends on cardiac output: if the heart cannot pump blood, oxygen cannot get to the tissues.

$$\text{Cardiac output} = \text{stroke volume} \times \text{heart rate}$$

From the above equation, you can see that cardiac output and blood pressure are dependent on the filling and emptying of the ventricles on every stroke (**stroke volume**), as well as on an adequate **heart rate.** An increase in heart rate can be tolerated as long as the ventricles can continue to completely fill. If the heart rate increase begins to affect ventricle filling, ventricle ejection is reduced, resulting in reduced blood pressure. Decreased blood pressure leads to **<u>hypoxia</u>** and, ultimately, shock.

Recognition of Shock

Sometimes the presence of shock may be obvious, whereas at other times you may need to depend on intuition (**Figure 5-2**). The best indicator for the presence of shock is the mechanism of injury (MOI). You should suspect that shock will develop if the MOI includes:

- Ejection from a moving vehicle
- Occupant death in the same passenger compartment
- Falls of greater than three times the patient's height
- Penetrating or **blunt trauma**
- Any condition associated with respiratory difficulty

If the patient is pale, cool, and clammy, it is shock until proven otherwise.

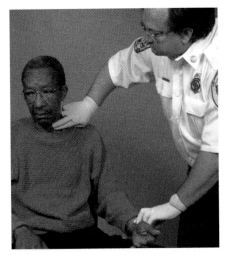

Figure 5-3 For a quick check of a patient's perfusion, compare the radial and carotid pulses at the same time.

Some important considerations to remember about patients in shock include:

- The majority of injured patients in shock are hypovolemic.

- **Cardiogenic** or **obstructive shock** may accompany any injury above the diaphragm.

- Closed head injuries *do not* cause shock. If the patient is hypotensive and has a closed head injury, assess him or her for bleeding.

- Septic shock is possible in patients if transport time from the scene is delayed.

Remember, in trauma cases, you should suspect shock even if the patient does not display shock symptoms.

Vital Signs

Changes in vital signs can indicate shock even before patient presentation begins to alter. Changes in blood pressure do not appear until 30% loss of total blood volume occurs. For a quick check of a patient's perfusion, feel for the presence of **radial** and **carotid pulses** at the same time and compare them (**Figure 5-3**). Use the following guidelines when comparing **central** and **peripheral pulses**.

- Carotid and radial pulses present indicate a systolic blood pressure of greater than 80 mm Hg

- Carotid with no radial pulse present indicates a systolic blood pressure of 60 to 80 mm Hg

- Carotid and radial pulses absent indicate a systolic blood pressure of less than 50 mm Hg—begin CPR

narrowing pulse pressure
The reduction of the gap between systolic and diastolic blood pressures, so that the systolic and diastolic numbers approach each other.

A **narrowing pulse pressure** indicates significant blood loss. Tachycardia can be another good indicator of the presence of shock. It is crucial to know tachycardia rates for different age groups. In beats per minute (BPM), tachycardia is defined as rates above:

- 100 BPM in adults

- 120 BPM in school-age children

- 140 BPM in toddlers

- 160 BPM in infants

Stages of Shock

Although there are many different levels of injury and systemic response, all shock can be categorized into one of three basic stages: the compensated stage, the progressive stage, and the irreversible stage.

Compensated Stage

In the **compensated stage** of shock, body defenses maintain adequate perfusion, and there are minimal outward signs of shock. The **sympathetic nervous system** responds to released epinephrine by helping the body maintain perfusion, but there are limits to the amount of compensation the body can provide. Here, fluid losses are minimal (usually less than 25% of total volume) and are usually replaced within 24 hours. Some signs include slight tachycardia, pallor, slightly narrowed pulse pressures, and delayed **capillary refill.**

Progressive Stage

As fluid losses continue, the body enters stage two of shock—the **progressive stage.** Fluid losses can be as high as 40% of total volume. In this stage the kidneys retain water to increase the circulating volume and release a very potent vasoconstrictor called **renin.** Renin further constricts **peripheral circulation** and effectively shuts down peripheral capillary beds, leading to the switch from **aerobic** to **anaerobic cellular respiration.** Acidosis begins to develop, and the body increases the respiratory rate to counteract the metabolic acidosis. Blood trapped in the extremities begins to show signs of **hypoxemia** (low oxygen concentrations in blood cells), causing cyanosis and **mottling.** The hypoxia and acidosis lead to decreased LOC. Decreased LOC, severe tachypnea, severe tachycardia, narrowed pulse pressures, and systemic cyanosis are the classic signs and symptoms of shock. However, if you wait for these to appear, you may begin treatment too late.

> **T**he classic signs and symptoms of shock appear in the progressive stage.

Irreversible Stage

If fluid loss and buildup of metabolic acids continue, the body can enter the **irreversible stage** of shock. In this stage, fluid losses are usually greater than 40% of total volume. The lack of oxygen leads to collapse of compensatory mechanisms. Circulating blood becomes toxic, and cellular damage becomes extensive. Cells rupture, releasing **lysosomes** that destroy tissue. The acidosis causes blood cells to become dysfunctional and misshapen, and they clog the capillary circulation by stacking up in a mechanism called **rouleaux formation.** All of these factors begin to affect the perfusion of vital organs (lungs, heart, brain, etc.), and the patient begins to undergo systems failure.

Types of Shock

Experts categorize shock into **actual fluid loss** and **perceived fluid loss.** In perceived fluid loss, fluid is displaced to another location in the body. Both perceived and actual fluid loss have the same signs and symptoms.

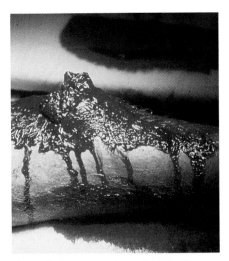

Figure 5-4 Hemorrhagic shock, a specific form of actual hypovolemia, results from actual blood loss.

Do not underestimate

the amount of fluid

that can be lost from perspiration.

Hypovolemic Shock

By definition, **hypovolemic shock** results when there is actual fluid loss from the body. The fluid losses can be from either water or blood. Using the pump/hoses/fluid analogy, you can think of hypovolemia as a fluid problem.

Actual Hypovolemia

Signs and symptoms of **actual hypovolemia** are directly related to the loss of circulating volume. Loss of circulating volume can result from either external or internal fluid losses.

External fluid losses can be due to several factors. One type of external fluid loss is GI loss, which can result from illness or exposures to any substance that can cause excessive vomiting or diarrhea, such as chemical substances like organophosphates. Both of these can lead to significant hypovolemias. Vomiting can induce metabolic alkalosis, whereas diarrhea can lead to metabolic acidosis.

Another type of external loss is perspiration. Water losses from sweating can exceed sodium losses and lead to an imbalance of salt and water. This imbalance leads to a condition called heat cramps and can evolve into the shock state of **heat exhaustion** if the fluid loss is not corrected.

A third type of external fluid loss, **diuresis**, can be caused by diuretic medications or by medical conditions such as diabetic ketoacidosis (DKA). Fluid loss from excessive urination can cause hypovolemia.

Internal losses are as significant as external losses but can be overlooked because they are hidden from view. Their effects can produce outward changes in a patient's presentation. Sources of internal fluid losses include inflammation and edema from infections or organ failure. Another source of internal loss, third spacing, is a result of the body's inability to retain fluid in the vascular compartment. The loss of blood proteins, tissue, or integrity of the vascular system leads to fluid shifting out of the vasculature. Conditions that predispose a patient to third spacing include burns, **peritonitis**, blunt trauma, and penetrating trauma.

Hemorrhagic Shock. A very specific form of actual hypovolemia that results from actual blood loss is hemorrhagic shock (**Figure 5-4**). Loss of blood is significant because it also depletes the oxygen-carrying capabilities and clotting factors of the blood—two essential defenses needed to counteract the developing shock. Hemorrhagic shock can be categorized into four phases (**see Table 5-1**). Note that the first signs and symptoms of shock do not appear until the patient is in the progressive phase.

When patients are unable to effectively communicate with others,

fluid loss is more likely to lead to significant hypovolemia.

Watch for hypovolemia in pediatric and geriatric patients.

Table 5-1. Phases of Hemorrhagic Shock

Category One—Compensated Phase	Characterized by: • Less than 15% of total blood volume lost, about 750 mL • Negligible changes in vital signs or LOC • Blood usually replaced by body within 24 hours

Category Two—Decompensated Phase	Characterized by:
	• Blood loss of 15% to 30%, or about 750 to 1,250 mL
	• Vital signs begin to indicate blood loss:
	  - Narrowing pulse pressures with developing postural hypotension
	  - First signs of altered LOC in the form of anxiety

Category Three—Progressive Phase	Characterized by:
	• Blood loss of 30% to 40%, or about 1,250 to 1,750 mL
	• Significant changes in vital signs:
	  - Tachycardia, tachypnea, hypotension
	  - Significantly altered LOC
	  - Pale, cool, clammy skin
	  - The first "obvious" signs and symptoms of shock appear

"The Bounce"	Metabolic attempt at perfusion restoration: • Release of enzymes and steroids that help restrict the vasculature and increase heart rate in order to increase perfusion • An ominous finding, it is a "last ditch" attempt by the body to restore perfusion; the patient appears to bounce back to normal

Category Four—Irreversible Phase	Characterized by:
	• Blood loss of greater than 40%, or more than 1,750 mL
	• Significant changes in vital signs:
	  - Unconscious, unresponsive
	  - Agonal respirations
	  - No blood pressure
	  - Mottled appearance to skin

Perceived Hypovolemia

Unlike actual hypovolemia, **perceived hypovolemia** is dilation of the vasculature, creating decreased circulating pressure and thus shock. In the pump/hoses/fluid analogy, perceived hypovolemia can be thought of as a hose problem. Vessels enlarge, allowing the circulating pressure to drop, creating the appearance of fluid loss by mimicking actual hypovolemia in patient presentation. Because the various types of perceived hypovolemia are associated with the poor distribution of fluids in the body, they can be grouped together and referred to as **distributive shock.** The four types of distributive shock are:

- **Neurogenic shock:** The inability of the central nervous system to communicate with the peripheral nervous system

- **Septic shock:** Overwhelming infections or cellular damage

> **P**erceived hypovolemias are associated with poor distribution of fluids in the body.

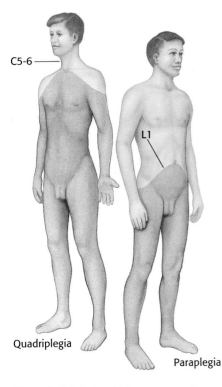

C5-6

L1

Quadriplegia

Paraplegia

Figure 5-5 Spinal cord injury can cause the loss of sympathetic tone beneath the site of injury.

- **Anaphylactic shock:** The overreaction of the immune system to a perceived threat
- **Obstructive shock:** Physical blockage of cardiac output
- **Cardiogenic shock:** Insufficient cardiac pumping

Neurogenic Shock. Neurogenic shock is the inability of the central nervous system to communicate with the peripheral nervous system. The spinal cord is a collection of continuous nerves that are bundled together in the spinal column. Nerves that exit the column first are usually layered on the outside of the bundle, whereas nerves that run the length of the column are layered toward the core of the bundle. Injury to the spinal cord can cause loss of **sympathetic tone** below the site of injury (**Figure 5-5**). Furthermore, the central nervous system loses the ability to communicate with the peripheral nervous system and thus cannot activate the systemic nervous system. This situation usually results from a traumatic injury to the spine. Complete trans-section of the spinal cord will result in complete paralysis of the body below the site of injury.

Signs and symptoms of neurogenic shock include:

- Above injury site, patient shows classic signs of shock, with pale, cool, and diaphoretic skin.
- Below site of injury, skin is pink, warm, and dry.
- Depending on the site of spinal injury, respiratory effort may be compromised.

Septic Shock. Septic shock is a type of shock that develops secondary to massive systemic illness or massive injuries. Patients in septic shock resulting from a bacterial infection usually are responding to toxic cellular breakdown of the microorganism, characterized by the release of endotoxins from bacterial destruction by the immune system or released exotoxins from the bacteria themselves. This cellular destruction leads to cellular hypoxia because the blood flow to organ capillary beds is disrupted, and ultimately leads to acidosis. As the cells begin dying, they burst, releasing their contents (**Figure 5-6**). If capillary **occlusions** last longer than 1 to 2 hours, organ damage becomes irreversible.

Signs and symptoms of metabolic sepsis include:

- High fever
- Severe weakness/patient is bedridden
- Recent history of illness
- Decreased LOC
- Hypotension
- Tachycardia
- Tachypnea
- Hot, flushed skin

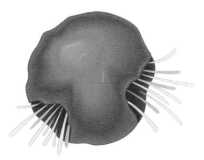

Figure 5-6 As cells begin dying, they burst and release their contents.

Anaphylactic Shock. Anaphylactic shock is a systemic overreaction of the immune system to an invading organism. The most common anaphylactic exposures result from antibiotics. Histamine dilates the vasculature at an infection site to allow the free movement of antibodies and macrophages into the infected area. With anaphylactic reactions, histamine is released systemwide, allowing fluid shifts into the tissues (**third spacing**) and creating potentially life-threatening edema. If this condition is not corrected, the third spacing can lead to shock, and the inflammation caused by the immune response can occlude the lower airways, where a majority of histamine receptors are found. Subcutaneous epinephrine and intravenous diphenhydramine hydrochloride (Benadryl) are the treatments of choice. Epinephrine constricts the vasculature and dilates the bronchioles, whereas diphenhydramine hydrochloride blocks the histamine receptors.

Signs and symptoms of anaphylactic shock include:

- Itching – mild to moderate
- Urticaria (hives) – mild to moderate
- Tachycardia – moderate to severe
- Tachypnea – moderate to severe
- Facial edema – severe
- Wheezing – severe
- Shortness of breath – severe
- Hypotension – severe

Obstructive Shock. Obstructive shock results from the physical blockage or impedance of cardiac function. Obstructive shock should be suspected in all cases of chest injuries above the diaphragm. In the pump/hoses/fluid analogy, obstructive shock can be though of as a pump problem. Conditions associated with obstructive shock are unique, as they do not often respond to fluid resuscitation, which increases the workload of the failing pump and could worsen the condition.

With obstructive shock often comes **tension pneumothorax**. Escaping air from punctured lung tissue begins to fill the potential space found between the **pleural linings**. As this space continues to fill, lung tissue is compressed and collapses (**Figure 5-7**). Trapped air increases until cardiac function is affected, thus acting like a **pericardial tamponade**.

third spacing
The shifting of fluid into the tissues, creating edema.

tension pneumothorax
An accumulation of air or gas in the **pleural cavity** that progressively increases and causes a rise in **intrathoracic pressure**.

pericardial tamponade
Acute compression of the heart due to a buildup of blood or other fluid in the pericardium.

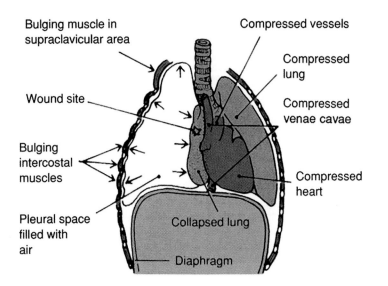

Bulging muscle in supraclavicular area

Compressed vessels

Compressed lung

Compressed venae cavae

Wound site

Bulging intercostal muscles

Compressed heart

Pleural space filled with air

Collapsed lung

Diaphragm

Figure 5-7 Tension pneumothorax.

Signs and symptoms of tension pneumothorax include:

- Decreased breath sounds on affected side
- Increasing shortness of breath (SOB)
- Tachycardia
- Tachypnea
- Asymmetrical chest movement
- **Hyperresonance** on affected side
- Hypotension

Pericardial tamponade results from either penetrating or blunt trauma to the chest. The **pericardium** is tough, fibrous, and difficult to penetrate, but the underlying heart is not. The **epicardium**, ventricles, and arteries of the heart can be lacerated by blunt or penetrating force even though the pericardium remains intact. When this happens, blood enters the pericardium, resulting in pressure on the heart, which prevents full ventricular filling and ejection. Decreased filling leads to decreased ejection, which in turn leads to decreased filling. The cycle continues until the patient experiences cardiac arrest.

Signs and symptoms of pericardial tamponade include:

- Muffled heart sounds
- Tachypnea
- Tachycardia
- Narrowing pulse pressures
- Distended jugular veins in sitting position

Cardiogenic Shock. Cardiogenic shock is defined as insufficient cardiac pumping due to cardiac damage or death. Leading causes of cardiogenic shock include acute myocardial infarction and myocardial contusion.

In **acute myocardial infarction,** if the infarct is large enough, cardiogenic shock can develop.

Signs and symptoms of cardiogenic shock or myocardial infarction include:

- Increasing SOB
- Ashen appearance
- Bradycardia
- Hypotension
- Chest pain

Myocardial contusion results from direct blunt trauma to the chest, bruising the surface of the heart and decreasing cardiac function (**Figure 5-8**). As with any bruise, inflammation and pain are results of the injury.

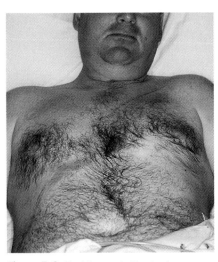

Figure 5-8 Blunt trauma to the chest.

Assessment of Shock

In order to manage any life-threatening condition, it is important not only to assess airway (A), breathing (B), and circulation (C), but also to recognize causes of ABC failure. This can be accomplished by following the ABC assessment model.

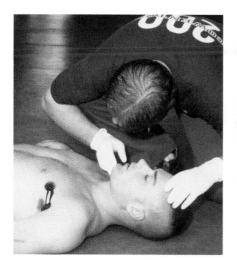

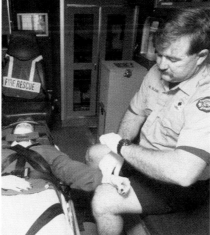

Figure 5-9 The respiratory pattern often reflects the adequacy of ventilation and may offer clues to the presence of shock.

Figure 5-10 The location of a palpable pulse may be a good indicator of systolic pressure.

When assessing for shock, begin by monitoring the ABCs for any problems that can be corrected. Follow with an assessment for the type of disability the patient is experiencing—for example, is it medical, trauma, neurogenic, or cardiogenic? Next, expose the patient to ensure you have covered everything in your assessment. For trauma patients, be prepared to expose the entire body. Be careful, respect privacy, and ensure adequate body heat retention, because all exposed skin loses heat quickly. Keep the assessment short.

Airway (A)

Your first concern should be the airway. An open airway is always necessary. Before any treatment to correct shock can take place, you must ensure an open airway.

Breathing (B)

Next, check the patient's breathing. After assessing the patient's airway status, ensure that there is proper ventilation. Evaluate the oxygen and carbon dioxide exchange by checking breath sounds, counting respirations, and observing the amount of effort needed for the patient to breathe (**Figure 5-9**). The respiratory pattern often reflects the adequacy of ventilation and may offer clues to the presence of shock. For example, if the patient is acidotic, respirations will be deep and rapid to help blow off carbon dioxide.

Circulation (C)

After you have checked the patient's airway and breathing, check circulation. You must control any serious bleeding first. You should suspect internal bleeding if the mechanism of injury (MOI) is present without external bleeding. Evaluate the patient's pulse for rate, quality, and location. A palpable peripheral pulse may be a good indicator of **systolic pressure** (**Figure 5-10**). One of the first changes noticed during the onset of shock is an increase in **pulse rate.**

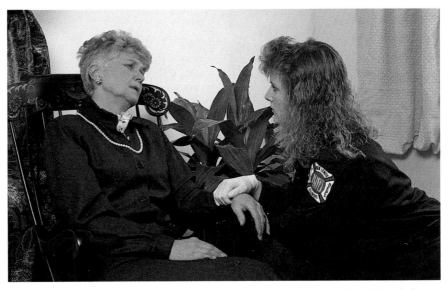

Figure 5-11 Evaluating a patient's LOC is important in determining the extent of cerebral perfusion.

Evaluation of skin color and temperature may be unreliable if the patient is in a hot or cold environment, or experiencing septic or neurogenic shock. Instead, pay attention to fingers, toes, and nose for cyanosis and delayed capillary refill times, even in adults. Treat internal bleeding with fluid replacement, high-flow oxygen, and possibly pneumatic anti-shock garments (PASG), depending on your protocols.

Further Assessment: Disability and Exposure

Evaluating the patient's LOC is important in determining the extent of cerebral perfusion (**Figure 5-11**). Possibly one of the best and earliest signs of impending shock is a change in LOC. As **cerebral ischemia** develops, the patient may become confused and agitated. You should consider any alteration of the patient's mental status a critical perfusion deficit. Assess the patient's LOC using the **AVPU scale** or the **Glasgow coma scale.**

Expose all the body surfaces to ensure that injuries are not hidden. This will also help you determine the mechanism of injury (**Figure 5-12**).

In summary:

- Suspect shock based on the mechanism of injury.

- Do not wait for the signs of shock to appear.

- Be on guard for shock with serious illness.

- Obtain as much patient information as possible and as much as the assessment will allow.

Treatment of Shock

Resuscitation of a patient in shock aims to restore adequate tissue perfusion as quickly as possible. In the event of hemorrhage,

cerebral ischemia
Poor blood flow through cerebral arteries due to some form of blockage or occlusion.

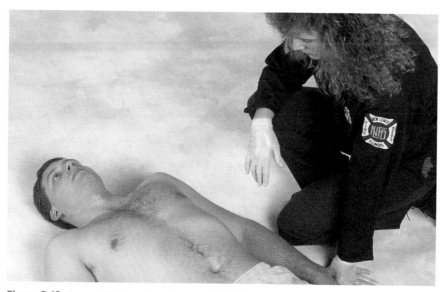

Figure 5-12 Expose all body surfaces to ensure that injuries are not hidden.

getting the patient to the proper medical facility for aggressive surgical intervention is critical. Fluid replacement, high-flow oxygen, and the possible use of PASG are critical for treatment.

External Hemorrhage—Actual Hypovolemias

In the case of external hemorrhaging, the potential for dying from uncontrolled bleeding is significant. Use direct pressure, elevation, and **pressure points** to control bleeding. PASG should be avoided, as they can cause clots to rupture, perpetuating the bleeding. Use IV fluids with caution because diluting the blood can lead to an induced anemia and exacerbate the hypoxia. Diluting blood also dilutes the clotting factors that help contain the bleeding. If fluid is needed to maintain the circulation, a good rule of thumb to remember is to infuse enough fluid to maintain a systolic pressure of 100 mm Hg.

Internal Hemorrhage—Actual Hypovolemias

The same potential exists for internal bleeding as does for external bleeding, except there are fewer options available to control bleeding. The risk of dying from uncontrolled bleeding is as prevalent here as in external hemorrhage, and thus the same precautions must be followed.

Nonhemorrhagic Shock—Perceived Hypovolemias

Perceived hypovolemia responds better to treatment with IV fluids and PASG than do other forms of shock. The exception is pericardial tamponade, which does not improve with either fluid or PASG resuscitation. Studies show that patients with this type of injury have a very high mortality rate, succumbing within 5 to 10 minutes from the onset of injury.

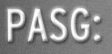

PASG:

Pneumatic Anti-Shock Garments

The Theory Behind the Use of PASG

It is thought that use of inflated pneumatic anti-shock garments (PASG)–sometimes called military anti-shock trousers (MAST)–aids in the treatment of patients in hemorrhagic shock by auto-transfusion (Figure 5-13). Blood from the lower extremities is, according to this theory, "transfused" back into the thorax and the core organs by compression of the vasculature in the lower extremities. In essence, PASG reduce the amount of hoses available for the blood to travel through by squeezing them shut. It is hoped that this shunting of blood will restore a perfusing blood pressure by increasing **peripheral vascular resistance (PVR).**

Although PVR is an important component in the maintenance of systemic blood pressure, increasing PVR leads to a decreased cardiac output, which is the opposite of what a patient who is bleeding needs. Increasing PVR can also rupture clots, leading to increased bleeding (Figure 5-14). Finally, once the PASG are deflated, trapped blood is allowed to re-enter the circulation, and patients can enter a state of instant acidosis. The use of PASG remains very controversial, and local protocols must be followed to ensure proper use.

Indications and Contraindications

PASG may be considered an effective tool for the treatment of circulatory collapse secondary to perceived hypovolemias such as:

- Septic shock
- Neurogenic shock
- Anaphylactic shock
- Extremity fractures or amputations
- Stabilization of femoral or pelvic fractures
- Cardiac arrest in which no pulses are generated by CPR

EMS systems usually establish their own protocols listing **contraindications,** but most agree that an **absolute contra-indication** to using PASG involves any compromise of breathing, as with pulmonary edema. The minute a patient shows signs and symptoms of any breathing difficulty, the use of PASG must be stopped immediately.

Relative contraindications to the use of PASG include:

- Cardiogenic shock
- Internal bleeding of the chest
- Impaled objects in the abdomen
- Third trimester of pregnancy
- **Evisceration**

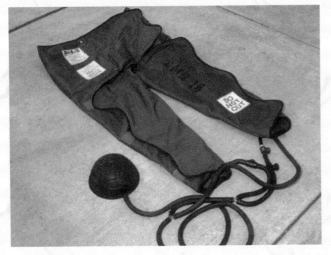

Figure 5-13 Pneumatic anti-shock garment.

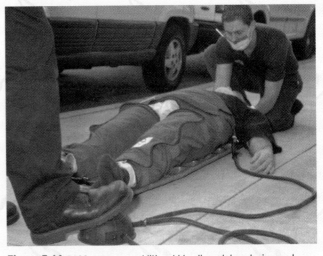

Figure 5-14 PASG can cause additional bleeding, clot rupturing, and acidosis. Therefore, PASG remain very controversial and local protocols must be followed to ensure proper use.

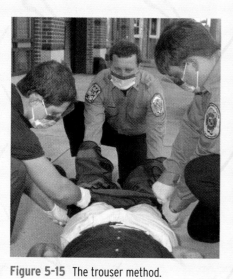

Figure 5-15 The trouser method.

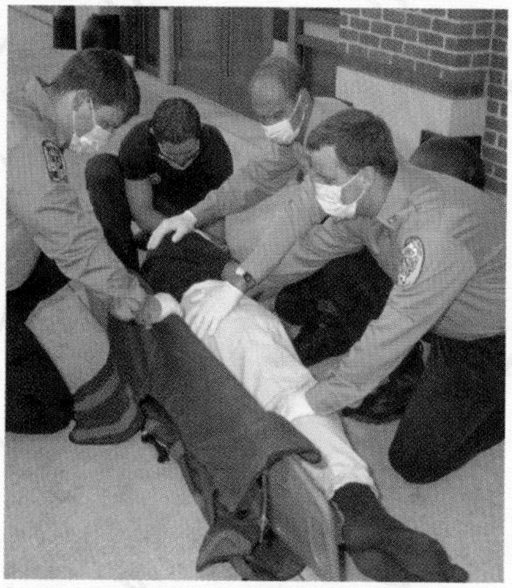

Figure 5-16 The logroll method.

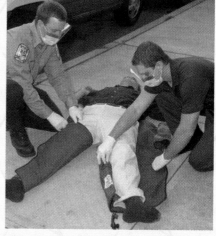

Figure 5-17 The diaper method.

Application

The decision to apply PASG should be based on the type of shock being experienced as well as the type of injury to the patient. For example, the use of PASG can make the use of other equipment—such as Hare traction splints, rigid splints, or bleeding control measures—cumbersome if not impossible. Possible application methods include:

- **Trouser method** (**Figure 5-15**): The PASG are applied as though they are a pair of pants. One EMT places his or her arms up through the PASG legs to grab the patient's ankles while the other EMTs help slide the PASG up over the patient.

- **Logroll method** (**Figure 5-16**): The PASG are placed on a backboard and the patient is logrolled onto the board and PASG. Once the patient is centered over the alignment markings of the PASG, the legs and abdomen are wrapped with the appropriate compartments and inflated according to protocol.

- **Diaper method** (**Figure 5-17**): The EMTs roll the inner edges and the anterior abdominal section of the PASG toward the center of the garment and then slide the pants underneath the patient, in the same way that they would slip a sheet underneath a patient. This method involves little movement of the patient and may be preferred when dealing with a hip injury.

Inflation

PASG should be used when the patient's systolic pressure falls below 100 mm Hg. The legs must be inflated individually before the abdominal portion is inflated. The stopcocks must be closed before inflation, with only one open at a time to fill the compartment. The compartments should be filled until either a systolic blood pressure of 100 mm Hg is reached or until the Velcro begins to pull apart.

Deflation

Deflation should rarely, if ever, be done in the prehospital setting, and then should be done only following a direct physician order. Before deflation takes place, the hospital needs to be able to correct the problem for which the PASG were initially used.

Wrap Up

Chapter 5
Causes and Treatment of Shock

Ready for Review

Shock results when the process of tissue perfusion is disrupted. This process can be disrupted when the heart provides inadequate pressure, when the vessels do not transport the fluid properly, or when the fluid itself does not provide adequate tissue perfusion. Because shock is often the result of fluid loss, it is obvious why IV therapy is a necessary treatment. Understanding the types of shock and the signs and symptoms will help you recognize shock and determine the best method of treatment for shock patients.

Quick Quiz

Answer each question below in your own words.

1) Describe the three main causes of shock in the body.

2) Describe the differences between actual and perceived hypovolemias.

3) List and briefly describe the types of perceived hypovolemias.

4) Should fluid resuscitation be used with obstructive shock? Why or why not?

5) Describe the difference in treatment modalities for external hemorrhagic, internal hemorrhagic, and nonhemorrhagic shock.

6) Discuss the theory behind the use of PASG.

7) A consequence of the use of PASG is the potential for cellular acidosis. Explain how cellular acidosis may occur.

8) List and discuss the applications when PASG would be indicated.

Altered Level of Consciousness

Regardless of the cause, patients with an **altered level of consciousness** will benefit from IV therapy. IV therapy is used not only to rehydrate these patients but also to provide access for medical treatment. A basic understanding of the causes of an altered LOC will help you make the correct decisions in IV therapy administration

AEIOU Tips

The patient who is experiencing an alteration in **mentation** can present a serious problem. There are several reasons for someone to have an altered level of consciousness. The following mnemonic is a simple way to remember them:

A-E-I-O-U-T-I-P-S

A	Alcohol
E	Epilepsy
I	Insulin
O	Overdoses
U	Uremia
T	Toxins/trauma
I	Infection
P	Psychologic disorders
S	Shock/stroke

Alcohol

Alcohol is a unique substance because it is so easily absorbed through the stomach **mucosa** directly into the blood. About 90% of consumed ethyl alcohol is metabolized in the liver, while the remainder is metabolized through the lungs, skin, and kidneys. Alcohol, in small doses, suppresses inhibitions. With chronic consumption, it is a central nervous system (CNS) depressant that impairs higher thought processes as well as motor functions. Consumption of large amounts of alcohol

> **A**lcohol abuse causes dehydration and impairment of higher thought processes and motor functions.

can cause diuresis by suppressing the production of antidiuretic hormone (ADH). Suppression of ADH allows the kidneys to release large amounts of water, leading to systemic dehydration.

There are two types of alcohol abuse:

- Chronic usage
- Acute usage

Patients with a history of chronic alcohol abuse show the effects of a lifetime of addiction and abuse. A generalized profile of this type of patient can include:

- Binge drinking episodes
- Blackouts
- Tremors in extremities
- Flushed skin
- **"Orange peel" nose**
- History of GI bleeding
- History of frequent accidents

Chronic alcohol abuse can lead to several disorders:

- Liver cirrhosis
- **Pancreatitis**
- **Esophageal varices**
- **Subdural hematoma**
- Hypoglycemia
- **Hepatic encephalopathy**

Signs and symptoms of acute alcohol abuse include:

- Strong smell of alcohol on breath
- Alcohol in contents of stomach
- Inability to maintain airway
- CNS depression
- Lethargy
- Coma
- Patient was in an environment where binge drinking occurred

An altered LOC is major concern when dealing with a patient who abuses alcohol and is experiencing **alcohol withdrawal syndrome** and alcohol-induced ketoacidosis. If a patient who abuses alcohol abruptly discontinues alcohol consumption, you may see the following symptoms:

- Noticeable tremors
- Possible seizures
- Nausea and vomiting
- Sweating
- Tachycardia

Alcohol-Induced Ketoacidosis

Alcohol consumption leads to poor nutritional habits. The anorexia and vomiting caused by alcohol abuse and the lack of carbohydrate intake lead to **ketoacidosis.** Systemic dehydration and depressed glucose synthesis in the liver lead to hypoglycemia and the use of fatty acids as an energy source. Alcohol metabolism also creates fatty acids that help contribute to the developing ketoacidosis.

ketoacidosis
An acidotic state created by the production of ketones via fat metabolism. See Chapter 4, "Principles of Fluid Balance" for an in-depth discussion of metabolic acidosis.

Acute Poisoning from Other Forms of Alcohol and Drugs

Often, patients who are alcohol-addicted will drink any form of alcohol to fulfill their desire. Common types of toxic alcohol include methanol, isopropyl alcohol, and ethylene glycol (**Figure 6-1**). Methanol is commonly referred to as wood grain alcohol and can cause blindness if consumed. Toxic amounts can be as little as 30 mL. Ethylene glycol is commonly found in antifreeze and does produce intoxication. Lethal doses can be as little as 100 mL.

Often, alcohol is not the only substance ingested. Recently, **date rape drugs** such as GHB (gamma hydroxybutyrate, also known as Georgia Home Boy, Grievous Bodily Harm, and Liquid Ecstasy) and Rohypnol (flunitrazepam, also known as Forget Me Drug, Lunch Money Drug, La Rocha, Forget Pill, Mexican Valium, Rocha Dos, Roofies, Roophies, Rope, Wolfies, Row Shay) have become more commonplace. In addition, drugs used to treat alcohol abuse withdrawal (for example, lorazepam [Ativan], diazepam [Valium], and clorazepate [Tranxene]) can become drugs of overdose (**Figure 6-2**).

IV access is often the only way that these acute poisonings can be managed. Antidotes (if available) need to be administered for certain drug overdoses, whereas alcohol poisonings require rehydration and medication.

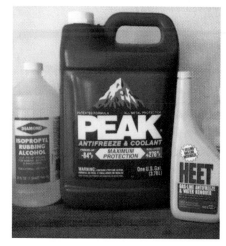

Figure 6-1 Common types of toxic alcohols.

Epilepsy

Seizures are associated with CNS dysfunction—not disease. This means that any illness or injury that has the ability to affect the CNS can cause a seizure. Seizures are often **idiopathic**—that is, there is no known medical reason for their development. The term **seizure disorder** is used to describe the syndrome of recurrent seizures without some underlying metabolic cause such as fever, diabetes, closed head injuries, etc.

Often seizures can be induced by several factors, such as:

- Hypoglycemia
- Drug overdose
- Hypoxia
- Alcohol
- Closed head injuries
- Cerebral bleeding

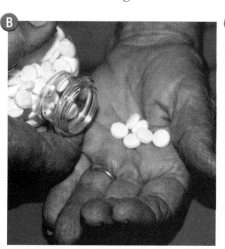
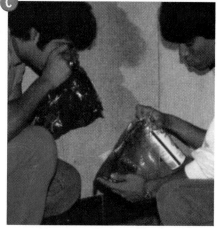

Figure 6-2 Some drug forms include injections, pills, and inhalants.

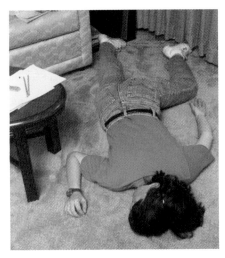

Figure 6-3 Following a grand mal seizure, the patient may enter the altered LOC postictal phase.

Persons with a seizure disorder can have seizure patterns that affect different areas of the brain and thus present in different ways. These types of seizures range from partial seizures that have a focal point of origin in the brain to **generalized seizures** that involve the entire brain. Partial seizures can be grouped into categories according to their effect on the patient.

Simple partial seizures do not affect consciousness but can affect areas of the brain controlling auditory, motor, or autonomic functions. **Jacksonian seizures,** which only affect one side of the body, are examples of simple partial seizures. In **complex partial** or **psychomotor seizures,** there may be some alteration in the patient's consciousness. These alterations may include **repetitive motor activity** like lip smacking or pill rolling of the fingers. You should also watch for hallucinations and psychotic behaviors, which are also common with these seizures.

Generalized seizures usually affect the entire brain and result in loss of consciousness. Generalized seizures can result in the "**daydream**" **seizure** (petit mal), in which the patient becomes flaccid and stares into space. These generalized seizures can also become the convulsive **tonic-clonic seizures** (grand mal) that are commonly associated with **epilepsy** (**Figure 6-3**). After a grand mal seizure, the patient may enter the altered LOC **postictal phase.** This is due to interruption of the **reticular activation system (RAS),** which collectively consists of the brainstem, pons, medulla, midbrain, hypothalamus, and thalamus, and its control over the conscious waking state of the brain.

Insulin

Insulin reactions manifesting in an altered LOC are the result of imbalances between insulin and glucose in the circulation. When mismatches between insulin and glucose occur, there are two possible consequences:

- Hypoglycemia from too little circulating glucose

- Hyperglycemia from too much circulating glucose

Regulation of glucose levels in the body is a complex and dynamic process that begins when absorbed carbohydrates stimulate the release of insulin from the **islets of Langerhans** beta cells in the pancreas. At that point, insulin mediates the transport of glucose across the cell membrane. The cells then convert the glucose and six oxygen molecules into 38 total adenosine triphosphate (ATP) molecules through processes that include **glycolysis** and the Krebs cycle. The use of oxygen means that this is aerobic metabolism, which creates carbon dioxide and water as by-products. The excess glucose is stored in the liver and skeletal muscles as glycogen. When blood glucose levels drop, the alpha cells of the islets of Langerhans release the hormone **glucagon** to convert the stored glycogen back into glucose through **gluconeogenesis.** If stored glycogen levels are depleted, the body will switch to fatty acid metabolism. In healthy endocrine systems, these shifts in metabolism are tolerated and never allowed to proceed to extremes.

Hypoglycemia

Hypoglycemia can be a problem in patients with diabetes who rely on daily injections of insulin (**Figure 6-4**). If insulin levels are not mediated by carbohydrate intake, imbalances between insulin and blood glucose levels form. Normal blood glucose levels range between 80 and 120 mg/dL. Hypoglycemia is defined as levels below 70 mg/dL, although symptoms may not be apparent in a patient until levels reach 60 mg/dL. Excess insulin depletes blood glucose levels, which stimulates the sympathetic nervous system to release epinephrine to restore blood glucose levels either by conversion of glycogen or the intake of carbohydrates.

Signs and symptoms of hypoglycemia include:

- Hunger
- Anxiety
- Sweating
- Vasoconstriction
- Tachycardia
- Hypotension
- Altered LOC

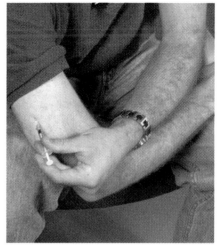

Figure 6-4 Hypoglycemia can be a problem in individuals with diabetes who rely on daily injections of insulin.

The brain gets its glucose without the aid of insulin because insulin cannot cross the blood-brain barrier, which regulates the substances allowed to cross into the cerebral circulation. Glucose can cross, but insulin cannot. Proper neurologic functions and the cellular metabolism of the brain rely on a certain amount of glucose being present in the cerebral circulation. If circulating blood glucose levels of the brain drop, neural cells begin to shut down, altering the patient's LOC. Because glucose is the fuel source for cellular metabolism, diminished cerebral glucose levels lead to the inability of the cells to use oxygen for aerobic cellular respiration. Cellular hypoxia develops, and the patient enters **insulin shock.** Signs and symptoms of developing hypoxia are:

hypoglycemia
Low circulating blood glucose levels.

- Pale, cool, clammy skin
- Altered LOC
- Cyanosis
- Tachycardia
- Tachypnea
- Hypotension

Signs and symptoms of insulin shock include:

- Headache
- Slurred speech
- Seizures
- Psychotic behavior
- Unconsciousness
- Coma

Treatment of Hypoglycemia: Dextrose 50% (D$_{50}$)

The treatment available for patients experiencing insulin-related problems is the administration of dextrose 50% (D$_{50}$) via IV. Remember to perform a blood glucose level check before you administer D$_{50}$ (**Figure 6-5**). It may be necessary to administer more than 1 amp of D$_{50}$ if the patient's blood glucose levels are extremely low or if the patient fails to respond fully to a single amp. Readminister D$_{50}$ in amounts according to local protocol if the patient does not become alert and oriented.

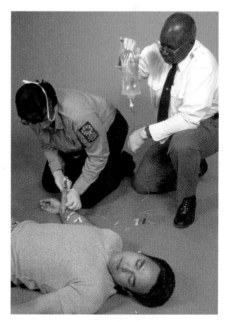

Figure 6-5 The treatment available for a patient who has insulin-related problems is administration of D$_{50}$ via IV.

Description and Indications. D_{50} is an IV medication used with patients who have hypoglycemia. It is usually supplied in ampoules containing 25 mg of dextrose dissolved in 50 mL of water.

Indications for use of D_{50} include:

- Symptomatic hypoglycemia

- Altered LOC for unknown reasons

- Unconsciousness with no obtainable patient history

- Medical cardiac arrest with a rhythm of **pulseless electrical activity (PEA)** or **asystole,** or with a history of diabetes

- **Glucometer** reading below 70 mg/dL

- Generalized **hypothermia**

Exercise caution when using D_{50}; contraindications include the presence of increased intercranial pressure or possible **intracranial bleeding.** A side effect of D_{50} is tissue **necrosis** and **phlebitis** with **extravasation.**

phlebitis
Inflammation of the vein.

necrosis
Cellular destruction resulting in tissue death.

Precautions. When administering D_{50}, take the following precautions:

- Check patient's blood glucose levels before you administer D_{50}, but do not rely on the accuracy of the glucometer reading. Consider the factors outlined on page 73 in "Patient Assessment and Treatment."

- Use caution with patients suspected of having low potassium levels, such as patients who are taking diuretics. Administering glucose in the presence of hypokalemia worsens the effects of low potassium. However, the potential for worsening the patient's hypokalemia should not be a factor when dealing with a truly hypoglycemic patient.

- Do not give oral glucose to a patient with an altered LOC.

Dosage. Dosages of D_{50} are as follows:

- Adult dose is a full amp of D_{50}.

- Children 3 months to 7 years old receive a full amp of D_{25} (empty half of an amp of D_{50} and draw up normal saline to fill the tube; this will give a concentration of 25%).

- Newborns to 3 months old receive D_{10} solution (put 2 mL of D_{50} into a syringe and add 8 mL of normal saline).

Administration. D_{50} is acidotic and will cause serious damage to tissue. You must give it by **IV push.** Follow the steps shown in **Box 6-1** to administer D_{50}.

Box 6-1:   Administration of D$_{50}$

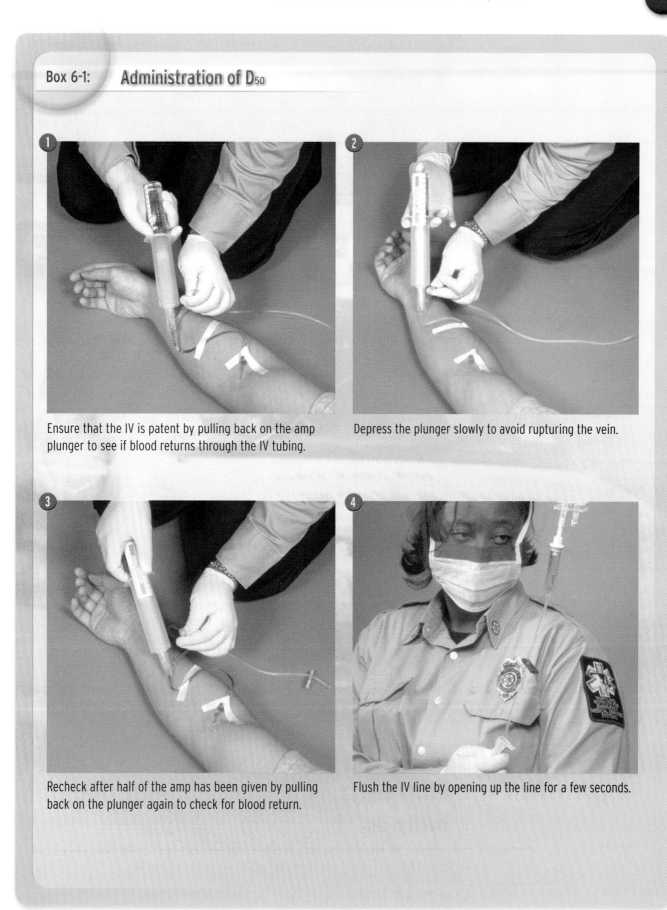

Ensure that the IV is patent by pulling back on the amp plunger to see if blood returns through the IV tubing.

Depress the plunger slowly to avoid rupturing the vein.

Recheck after half of the amp has been given by pulling back on the plunger again to check for blood return.

Flush the IV line by opening up the line for a few seconds.

Stimulants can create a state of paranoia and can place the patient at risk of cardiac arrest due to excessive stimulation of the autonomic nervous system. Depressants suppress the patient's response to stress, stimulation, and pain, and block the autonomic nervous system which regulates the body's involuntary functions.

Hyperglycemia

hyperglycemia
High circulating blood glucose levels.

Hyperglycemia, or high circulating blood glucose levels, occurs when a person ingests a large amount of carbohydrates, such as a large pasta dinner. Normally, high carbohydrate levels are tolerated and returned to normal through metabolic pathways. Problems arise when blood glucose levels remain elevated and cannot be corrected. Hyperglycemia (blood glucose levels greater than 250 mg/dL) and its side effects (diuresis, electrolyte losses) create metabolic acidosis. People most at risk for hyperglycemia are patients with insulin-dependent diabetes. If a person with diabetes neglects to regulate insulin/glucose levels closely, glucose begins to accumulate in the extracellular compartments. The cells switch to fatty acid metabolism, which leads to the production of ketoacids, increasing the developing metabolic acidosis. Remember that with metabolic acidosis, the compensatory mechanism is the respiratory system. The patient may become tachypnic in order to blow off the excess ketoacids, and begin rapid, deep **Kussmaul respirations.** Patients who have developed ketoacidosis present with a fruity breath odor, often mistaken for alcohol intoxication, because it can smell like the patient has been drinking wine.

Signs and symptoms to watch for in patients with diabetic ketoacidosis can be categorized by the stage of the illness. During the initial phases, signs and symptoms are related to the diuresis:

- Warm, flushed skin
- Tachycardia
- Hypotension
- Weak pulses

With the development of ketoacidosis, signs and symptoms include:

- Nausea and vomiting
- Anorexia
- Ketone (fruity) odor on breath
- Lethargy
- Abdominal pain
- Coma

Overdoses

Accidental or intentional drug overdoses can appear in patients of any age. Drugs can be categorized into two basic types:

- Stimulants
- Depressants

Stimulants work by stimulating the sympathetic nervous system and causing a massive release of epinephrine, or an **epi dump.** The danger with stimulants is the possibility of overstimulation of the **sympathetic response.** Stimulants such as lysergic acid diethylamide (also known as acid or LSD), phenycyclidine (PCP), and psilocybin mushrooms can create a state of paranoia, making some patients difficult to manage. Other drugs of this type, such as cocaine, crack, and crystal metham-phetamines (ice) can place the patient at risk of cardiac arrest from drug-induced **tachyarrhythmias.**

Depressants work by depressing the sympathetic response, usually by blocking the **autonomic nervous system,** which regulates the automatic functions of the body such as the respiratory system and heart function. **Barbiturates** (such as phenobarbital), tranquilizers (such as diazepam), and **narcotics** (such as codeine, morphine, and heroin) all suppress the patient's response to stress and/or stimulation. Pain is considered a stressor and a stimulant for sympathetic stimulation.

Overdose Management

A patient can overdose on street drugs as well as on those prescribed by physicians. It is very important that you make every effort to identify the drug involved, because the treatment for different drugs can vary greatly. Look for evidence of empty bottles, needles, unidentified para-phernalia, etc. Some examples of the varying treatments for different drugs, including stimulants, depressants, and other drugs that do not fit into either of these categories (such as acetaminophen), are listed below.

- *Heroin, opiate, and synthetic opiate overdoses* require immediate airway maintenance and IV naloxone hydrochloride (Narcan). Naloxone hydrochloride has become a commonly used treatment in the prehospital setting and emergency department. Some things to know about naloxone hydrochloride include:

  - Naloxone hydrochloride is a competitive inhibitor used to block binding of opiates to their associated receptor sites in the CNS, effectively reversing the overdose.

  - The **half-life** of naloxone hydrochloride is considerably shorter than that of opiates or narcotics, creating the need for repeat dosing to maintain the patient's LOC.

  - The effects of naloxone hydrochloride are almost instantaneous and can create a hostile patient when the person is aroused from the narcotic state.

  - Rapid IV push can lead to overstimulation of the sympathetic nervous system, and the patient may vomit, sometimes violently.

  - Naloxone hydrochloride is only effective on overdoses of opiates (morphine, codeine) and "opiate-like" compounds such as meperidine hydrochloride (Demerol) and heroin.

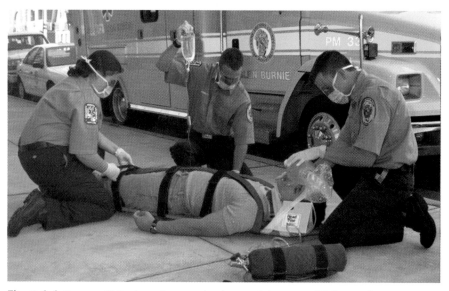

Figure 6-6 Diazepam (Valium) overdoses require airway maintenance and IV flumazenil.

- *Diazepam (Valium) overdoses* require airway maintenance and IV flumazenil (Romazicon) (**Figure 6-6**). Flumazenil works much the same way as naloxone hydrochloride; it is specific for diazepam (Valium), and its patient response is similar to that of naloxone hydrochloride.

- *Tricyclic overdoses* require constant cardiac monitoring as life-threatening arrhythmias can and do occur rapidly; IV sodium bicarbonate is also used to counteract the **cardiotoxic** effects of **tricyclics** (**Figure 6-7**).

- *Acetaminophen overdoses* require acetylcysteine, though medical control may order **activated charcoal.**

- *Cocaine overdoses* require cardiac monitoring as arrhythmias occur and may ultimately require treatment and IV morphine administration to block the stimulation of the sympathetic nervous system.

Uremia

Kidney failure causes retention of uremic toxins and leads to the development of **uremic encephalopathy.** Patients experience altered LOCs, followed by an inability to identify objects and people. Eventually, patients develop delirium and become stuporous and comatose.

As an EMT, if you encounter a patient with **uremia,** he or she will undoubtedly be a renal patient. These patients may be from a dialysis center or home care, or you may encounter them during an interfacility transport. There is little if any treatment you can provide other than to obtain a patient history, perform a patient assessment for mentation and hydration (see "Patient Assessment and Treatment" on page 73), and initiate IV access (or maintain an established IV). If IV access is required, you must restrict it to the extremity without an **arteriovenous shunt** (dialysis shunt) in place. These shunts are used in the blood filtering process and can be found either outside the body or inside (an internal shunt can be surgically created by linking an artery and a vein in the underlying vasculature of the arm or the leg for easier dialysis access).

> **T**reatment of uremia patients includes obtaining a patient history, performing an assessment, and initiating IV access.

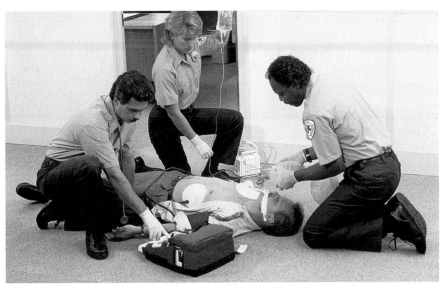

Figure 6-7 Tricyclic overdoses require constant cardiac monitoring.

These shunts pose a great risk of hemorrhage if they are used inappropriately. It would be unwise to administer high amounts of fluid to patients with kidney failure because this could lead to circulatory overload.

Toxins/Trauma

Toxins

Toxins and poisons interfere with biological functions of the body. Exotoxins are proteins released during the growth of the bacterial cell and can produce vomiting and diarrhea. Neural toxins work by binding to neural synapses and preventing the release or reabsorption of neural transmitters, thereby causing paralysis. Blocking of neural transmission can have dire consequences if the affected neural pathway is to the lungs, heart, or other vital muscle mass of the body.

Animal and insect venoms target different tissues. Most animal toxins (such as venom from snakebites) slow down or paralyze the victim by blocking the release of neural transmitters, making the intended food source easy to catch and eat (**Figure 6-8**). Insect toxins (such as venom from spider bites) are protein-dissolving toxins that create a "protein soup" of the prey, making the food source easy to digest (**Figure 6-9**).

Toxins and poisons also include chemical compounds. Several organic and inorganic compounds can poison the patient and create an altered LOC. Sometimes poisonings occur after an attempt by the patient to use the toxic compound as a drug, as is often the case with **huffers**—people who inhale fumes from any petroleum distillant such as solvents found in paint, gasoline, and glue. Sometimes the poisonings are accidental, as with exposure to **organophosphates** used as insecticides.

Poisonous and/or toxic compounds can be introduced into a patient by:

- Ingestion
- Absorption
- Inhalation
- Injection

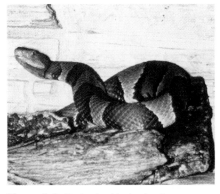

Figure 6-8 Most animal toxins (such as venom from snakebites) are intended to slow down or paralyze the victim by blocking the release of neural transmitters.

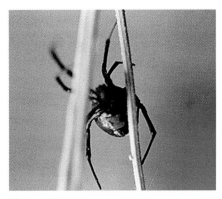

Figure 6-9 Insect toxins (such as venom from spider bites) are protein-dissolving toxins, intended to create a "protein soup" of the prey.

There are limited treatment options available for toxins. Management consists of maintaining vital functions (either by manual ventilation or CPR, as shown in **Figures 6-10 and 6-11**) and IV access (direct vascular access for drug administration is crucial).

Trauma

Trauma can lead to an altered LOC in many different ways. For example, hypovolemia leads to decreased cerebral perfusion and an altered LOC. The goal is to restore the circulating volume and the control of the body by the brain. Hemorrhage, like hypovolemia, leads to an altered LOC through decreased cerebral perfusion. The key difference is that hemorrhage involves a loss of oxygen-carrying capabilities because of the loss of blood; IV fluid replacement is only a temporary fix.

Closed Head Injury. **Closed head injury** can lead to an altered LOC as brain tissue swells in the cranium. The most serious closed head injury is one that causes bleeding into the cranium.

Epidural bleeding develops when trauma to the head causes shearing and tearing of the arteries that enter the brain tissue from above the dural linings. This rapidly developing life-threatening injury is characterized by a suspected loss of consciousness episode followed almost immediately by a conscious, altered "lucid" interval. This interval is followed by a gradually deteriorating LOC, unconsciousness, seizures, and death.

Subdural bleeding is venous bleeding that develops more slowly than epidural bleeding but is just as dangerous. Subdural bleeding is slower, and develops beneath the dural coverings of the brain. Subdural bleeding is associated with both traumatic and nontraumatic injuries. The patient presents with a gradual deterioration in LOC that developed over hours or sometimes days. Patients become unresponsive and die from the effects of the bleeding. Anyone who has an altered LOC should be evaluated for bleeding.

Patients with a serious closed head injury can present with any of the following:

- Increased blood pressure to overcome the increasing intracranial pressure

- Decreased pulse rate to allow the ventricles to fill and eject the most pressure

- Changes in respiratory pattern reflecting the infarction of the brainstem as a result of increasing intracranial pressure.

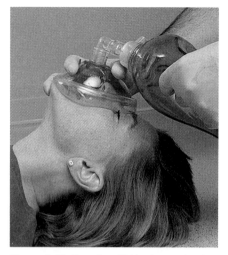

Figure 6-10 Manual ventilation is a method for maintaining vital functions.

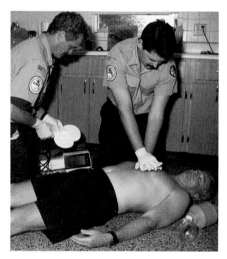

Figure 6-11 Administering CPR helps to maintain vital functions.

> **T**hough epidural and subdural bleeding develop at different rates, both can be fatal. A patient with an altered LOC must always be evaluated for bleeding.

A Brief Word About Closed Head Injuries and Artificial Ventilations

Injury to the brain from trauma can result in increasing intracranial pressure from bleeding or edema, and possibly in pressure on the brainstem, which can affect respiratory rate. The edema begins to collapse cerebral circulation, leading to acidosis of brain cells. The compensatory mechanism for this acidosis is tachypnea, as evidenced by the increasing respiratory rate of patients with closed head injuries.

If you have not thoroughly assessed the mechanism for the patient's hyperventilation, you may misinterpret these signs as anxiety-induced hyperventilation and attempt to treat the patient by slowing down his or her breathing and withholding oxygen. Or, you may recognize the reason for hyperventilation as the closed head injury and begin treatment by increasing the hyperventilation to further reduce the cerebral edema.

Either of these treatment plans could lead to deterioration of the patient's condition from acid/base imbalances. Increasing the respiratory rate leads to respiratory alkalosis and hypercalcemia, causing vasoconstriction of cerebral vasculature. This vasoconstriction leads to diminished blood flow to the areas of the brain that desperately need oxygen in the first place to reduce the developing acidosis.

When ventilating a closed head injury patient, you need to focus on moderate hyperventilation specific to the age group (just enough to reduce the cerebral acidosis but not so much that you create cerebral alkalosis). The use of end tidal carbon dioxide detectors is useful in determining the amount of expired carbon dioxide to help assess the adequacy of ventilation.

Infection

Infection and <u>sepsis</u> can lead to an altered LOC. It is important to remember the difference between an infection and sepsis. Infections tend to be localized and for the most part contained, whereas **sepsis** refers either to an infection that has spread to other areas of the body or to multiple infections occurring at the same time. An altered LOC can be caused by:

- Elevated body temperature
- Sepsis
- Toxins released by the bacteria, virus, or fungus causing the infection

The more advanced the infection or sepsis, the more likely the patient will exhibit signs of an altered LOC. Some presentations of altered LOC can be difficult to unravel. For example, the altered LOC of a respiratory infection may result from either the inefficient oxygen/carbon dioxide exchange or the sepsis created by the infection. When a patient does become septic, the circulating toxins can cause extreme disorientation and confusion. IV access is critical for the patient to facilitate rehydration and provide access for antibiotics (**Figure 6-12**). Often, simple rehydration can greatly improve a patient's LOC.

sepsis
(1) An infection that has spread to other areas of the body; (2) multiple infections occurring at the same time; (3) reaction to the spilled contents of destroyed cells, as seen with crushed tissue and organs.

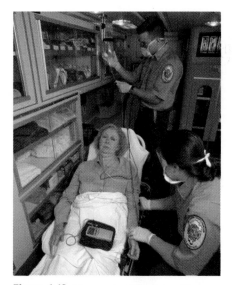

Figure 6-12 IV access is critical for septic patients in order to facilitate rehydration and provide access for antibiotics.

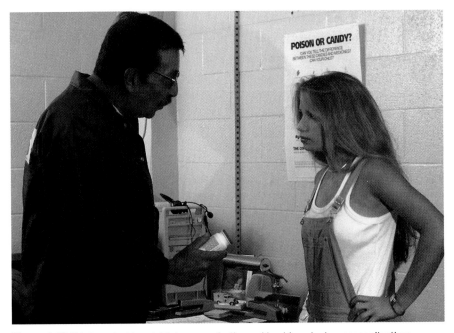

Figure 6-13 It is important to establish communication and trust in order to manage situations involving psychologic problems.

Psychologic Disorders

There is often confusion between psychologic disorders and behavior disorders. Behavior disorders are usually a consequence of the patient's inability to deal with or function in a given situation. Stress can cause the patient to act out, be unaware of his or her actions, and/or have no understanding of the circumstances. Managing this type of situation should include acknowledging the patient's concerns; removing him or her from the area; trying to get him or her to refocus on the situation; and establishing boundaries by indicating what behavior is acceptable and what is not. This will aid in ensuring the safety of the patient, yourself, and your partner. Above all, try to be patient.

Psychologic disorders have an underlying pathophysiology that can make dealing with this type of patient difficult. It is very important that you attempt to establish some type of communication and trust to manage the situation (**Figure 6-13**). Make every attempt to identify the nature of the patient's problem: identify the patient's history, any medications taken or missed, the events that precipitated the crisis, and any other information relevant to the patient's current crisis.

With both behavior and psychologic emergencies, keep your patient care management simple, and you will be able to ease the situation greatly. Remember that your personal safety comes first—never enter a place you cannot safely leave.

Shock/Stroke

Shock can lead to an altered LOC, as discussed in previous chapters. It is critical to remember that an altered LOC associated with shock is a serious sign: it means that brain perfusion is decreasing. Once this happens, other defense mechanisms begin to fail.

Patients who have had a stroke or cerebrovascular accident (CVA) present with an altered LOC. There are basically two types of CVAs:

- *Intravascular blockage (brain attack)* occurs as a result of either blood clots or **plaque** buildup. These types of CVAs are often called ischemic cerebrovascular accidents.

- *Vascular rupture* (usually arterial) allows blood to leave the vascular space and damage brain tissue.

Intravascular blockage results in brain tissue being deprived of oxygen and becoming **ischemic,** much like a heart attack. As with a heart attack, ischemic brain tissue will infarct, and sensory loss may become permanent. New medical technology has provided a treatment for this type of CVA that is very similar to the clot-busting treatment given to heart attack patients.

Vascular rupture can result from:

- Trauma causing epidural, subdural, or intracerebral bleeding

- Medical reasons such as high blood pressure and/or hardening (and thus weakening) of the cerebral arteries

- A genetically weakened area of circulation that is predisposed to an **aneurysm**

Vascular bleeding can arise from both nontraumatic and traumatic reasons. Combative behavior can be common for patients experiencing traumatic bleeding, making patient management difficult. For years, the standard of treatment for "brain swelling" from a closed head injury included hyperventilation. However, hyperventilation can lead to decreased perfusion to all brain tissue, increasing the ischemia. To avoid this, ventilate these patients at slightly elevated levels. Current treatment for suspected CVAs mirrors the treatment for acute myocardial infarctions (AMIs): **thrombolytics.** It is imperative that any patient suspected of suffering from a CVA be quickly diagnosed and transported to a facility that can administer treatment, as the treatment window for ischemic CVAs is dangerously small.

> **V**entilate stroke patients at slightly elevated levels.

Patient Assessment and Treatment

Often patients will present with an altered LOC without any available history. It is your role as the EMT to find clues that indicate the potential cause for the altered LOC. Your overall patient assessment should include a focus on events that led up to the crisis:

- Were alcohol, overdose, or trauma involved?

- Is there any history that would support a diagnosis of epilepsy, hypoglycemia, infection, psychologic disorder, or stroke?

- Is there evidence that suggests uremia, toxins, or shock?

- Is the patient's presentation and affect normal? (Ask caretakers or family.)

- What events precipitated the change in the patient's LOC?

- When did this episode start and how long has it continued?

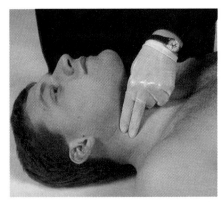

Figure 6-14 Circulation assessment should include checking pulse quality, irregularities, and rate.

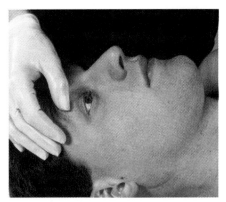

Figure 6-15 Eyes should be assessed for pupillary response.

The physical assessment of the patient with an altered LOC must be more thorough than with other patients, as patient and event histories are probably going to be difficult to obtain. A complete patient assessment is often critical for proper diagnosis of a patient with an altered LOC:

- *Skin assessment* should include checking for color, condition, and injection or puncture marks.

- *Circulation assessment* should include assessing pulse quality, irregularities, and rate (**Figure 6-14**).

- *Respiratory assessment* should include breath sound quality, rate, fluid buildup, and possible obstructions.

- *Eye assessment* should include **pupillary response** (**Figure 6-15**). Constricted pupils indicate **parasympathetic stimulation,** often associated with depressants, narcotics, etc. Dilated pupils are often a sign of sympathetic stimulation, associated with cocaine, methamphetamines, LSD, etc.

Treatment for patients with an altered LOC involves:

- Assessing and maintaining ABCs

- Administering high-flow oxygen

- Establishing IV access

- Communicating with the patient (if possible)

- Determining the patient's condition (stable or deteriorating)

- Providing rapid transport in case the patient can be treated with medication

- Treating any associated injuries

- Considering antidotes, if applicable:
  - Activated charcoal
  - **Syrup of ipecac**
  - Glucose
  - Fluids
  - Oxygen

Wrap Up

Chapter 6
Altered Level of Consciousness

Ready for Review

When dealing with patients with an altered LOC, remember the causes: Alcohol, Epilepsy, Insulin, Overdoses, Uremia, Toxins/trauma, Infections, Psychologic disorders, and Shock/stroke. Knowing the signs and symptoms that correspond to these causes will assist you in administering the correct IV fluid in the appropriate quantity.

Quick Quiz

Answer each question below in your own words.

1 Describe the process of insulin shock.

_____

2 List and briefly describe three of the possible medical complications associated with chronic alcohol abuse.

_____

3 Describe the differences between hypoglycemia and DKA.

_____

4 List and explain the different patient presentations expected with the use of stimulants and depressants.

_____

5 Describe what naloxone hydrochloride is used for and how it works.

_____

6 Explain the management techniques for dealing with a patient who presents with a behavior disorder.

_____

7 List and describe the different types of cerebral vascular accidents.

_____

8 List the information an EMT needs to treat a patient who has an altered LOC of unknown origin.

_____

9 How does uremia lead to an altered LOC?

_____

Chapter 7

IV Techniques and Administration

The most important thing to remember about IV techniques and fluid administration is to keep the intravenous equipment sterile. Forethought will help prevent mental and procedural errors while starting the IV.

One way to ensure proper technique is to develop a routine to follow as you assemble the appropriate equipment. A routine will help you keep track of your equipment and the steps necessary to complete a successful IV.

Assembling Your Equipment

To avoid delays or the possibility of IV site contamination, gather and prepare all your equipment before you attempt to start an IV. Sometimes the condition and presentation of the patient make full preparation difficult. This is where working as a team becomes critical. It is often the members of your own crew who, by anticipating your needs, help make the IV equipment assembly possible. **Box 7-1** shows a logical sequence of steps in assembling your equipment; each will be described in this chapter.

Choosing an IV Solution

Prehospital patient care and IV therapy center on identifying the type of situation and the needs of the patient. Ask yourself:

- Is the patient a trauma patient?
- Is the patient a medical patient?
- Does the patient need fluid replacement?

In the prehospital setting, the choice of IV solution is limited to the **isotonic crystalloids** normal saline and lactated Ringer's solution. D_5W (5% dextrose in water) is often reserved for administering medication because the presence of dextrose has the potential to alter fluid and electrolyte levels in the body.

Box 7-1:   Steps in Assembling IV Equipment

1. Get your gloves on! BSI cannot be emphasized strongly enough.
2. Choose a solution—check the bag for clarity, expiration, and correct solution.
3. Choose an administration set appropriate for the patient and the needs of the patient.
4. Choose an appropriate IV site.
5. Choose an appropriately sized catheter.
6. Recheck your work before you go any further.
7. Tear tape for securing the IV site.
8. Have blood tubes close by.
9. Set up the Luer adapter and the Vacutainer barrel, or have a syringe close by for drawing blood.
10. Have a couple of catheters ready for insertion.
11. Open an alcohol wipe.
12. Have 4" x 4" pieces of gauze ready for catching blood.
13. Then, and only then, apply a constricting band (it is the last thing done before inserting the IV).
14. Insert the catheter and complete your blood draws.
15. Hook up the IV tubing and adjust the flow.
16. Secure the site and the blood tubes.
17. Administer medication if necessary.
18. Adequately dispose of sharps.
19. Document everything you did.

Each IV solution bag is wrapped in a protective sterile plastic bag and is guaranteed to remain sterile until the posted expiration date. Once the protective wrap is torn and removed, the IV solution has a shelf life of 24 hours. The bottom of each IV bag has two ports: an injection port for medication, and an **access port** for connecting the administration set. The sterile access port is protected by a removable pigtail that represents a point-of-no-return line—once this pigtail is removed, the bag must be used immediately or discarded.

IV solution bags come in different fluid volumes (**Figure 7-1**). Volumes commonly used in hospitals are 1,000 mL, 500 mL, 250 mL, and 100 mL; the more common prehospital volumes are 1,000 mL and 500 mL. The smaller volumes (250 mL and 100 mL) more commonly contain D_5W and are used for mixing and administering medication via IV **"piggyback"** administration.

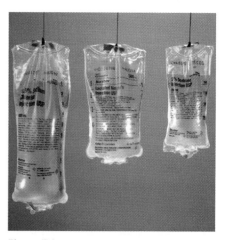

Figure 7-1 Examples of different IV bag sizes.

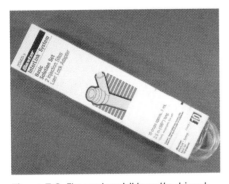

Figure 7-2 The number visible on the drip set refers to the number of drops it takes for a milliliter of fluid to pass through the orifice and into the drip chamber.

Choosing an Administration Set

An **administration set** moves fluid from the IV bag into the patient's vascular system. As with IV solution bags, IV administration sets are sterile as long as they remain in their protective packaging. Once they are removed from the packaging, their sterility cannot be guaranteed. Each IV administration set has a **piercing spike** protected by a plastic cover. Again, once the piercing spike is exposed and the seal surrounding the cap is broken, the set must be used immediately or discarded.

There are different sizes of administration sets for different situations and patients. Most **drip sets** have a number visible on the package (**Figure 7-2**), which indicates the number of drops it takes for a milliliter of fluid to pass through the orifice and into the **drip chamber.** Drip sets come in two primary sizes: microdrip and macrodrip. **Microdrip sets** allow 60 **gtt** (drops)/mL through the small, needlelike orifice inside the drip chamber. Microdrips are ideal for medication administration or pediatric fluid delivery because it is easy to control their fluid flow. **Macrodrip sets** allow 10 to 15 gtt/mL through a large opening between the piercing spike and the drip chamber. Macrodrip sets are best used for rapid fluid replacement but can also be used for maintenance and **keep-the-vein-open (KVO) IV set-ups.**

Blood tubing or **blood pumps** are special types of macrodrip sets designed to facilitate rapid fluid replacement by **manual infusion** of either multiple IV bags or IV/blood replacement combinations. Most pumps have dual piercing spikes that allow two bags of fluid to be hung at once on the same patient (**Figure 7-3**). The central drip chamber has a special filter designed to filter the blood during infusions.

Preparing an Administration Set

After choosing the IV administration set and the IV solution bag, verify the expiration date of the solution and check for solution clarity. Prepare to spike the bag with the administration set as indicated in **Box 7-2**.

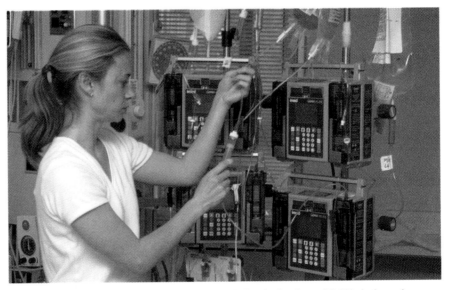

Figure 7-3 Most pumps have dual piercing spikes that allow for two bags of fluid to be hung at once on the same patient.

Box 7-2:   Spiking the Bag

Remove the rubber pigtail found on the end of the IV bag by pulling on it. The bag is still sealed and will not leak until the piercing spike of the IV punctures this port.

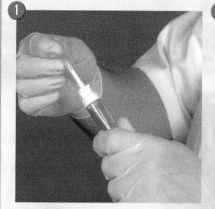

Remove the protective cover from the piercing spike (remember, this spike is sterile!).

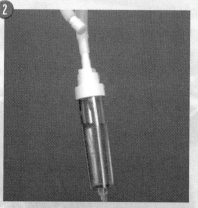

Slide the spike into the IV bag port until you see fluid enter the drip chamber.

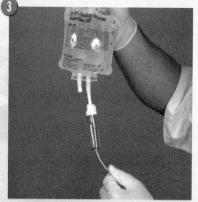

Allow the solution to run freely through the drip chamber and into the tubing to prime the line and flush the air out of the tubing.

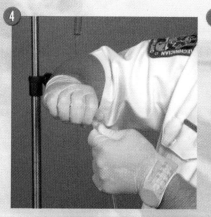

Twist the protective cover on the opposite end of the IV tubing to allow air to escape. Do not remove this cover yet, because the cover keeps the tubing end sterile until it is needed. Let the fluid flow until air bubbles are removed from the line before turning the roller clamp wheel to stop the flow.

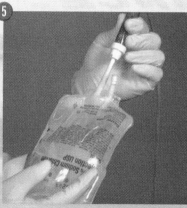

Next, go back and check the drip chamber; it should be only half filled. The fluid level must be visible to calculate drip rates. If the fluid level is too low, squeeze the chamber until it fills; if the chamber is too full, invert the bag and the chamber and squeeze the chamber to empty the fluid back into the bag.

Hang the bag in an appropriate location with the end of the IV tubing easily accessible.

Box 7-3:   **Assembly of the Blood Pump**

- Choose one of the two spikes present. Often, but not always, these spikes are different colors, one red and one white. Usually, the red spike is used for blood administration unless two IV bags are needed for the patient.

- Invert the pump to prime the line. IV fluid forces all of the air out of the pump so it can function properly. Keep the pump lower than the drip chamber to fill it: hold the IV bag high in one hand and let the IV set hang from the bottom of the bag; grab the pump with the other hand and invert it, so that the fluid enters and fills the pump *from the bottom up*. Once the pump is filled, you can release it and let it hang normally.

- Make sure the fluid level inside the drip chamber covers the filter completely prior to administration of blood. This will help prevent blood cells from rupturing as they pass through the filter (**Figure 7-4**).

- Watch flows closely, because the filters of a blood pump can quickly become clogged.

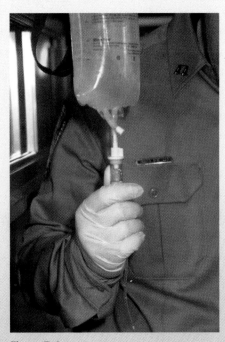

Figure 7-4 The fluid level inside the drip chamber must cover the filter completely prior to administration of blood.

Assembling and filling blood pumps (sometimes called a trauma setup) can be difficult if you are not familiar with the operation. Priming the line and the pump must be accomplished in a specific manner. The pump must be void of any air to work properly. **Box 7-3** indicates how to assemble a blood pump.

Choosing an IV Site

It is important to select the most appropriate vein for IV catheter insertion. Avoid areas of the vein that contain valves because a catheter will not pass through these areas easily and the needle will cause damage. Valves can be recognized as small bumps located in the vein. Use the following criteria to select a vein:

- Locate the vein section with the straightest appearance.
- Choose a vein that has a firm, round appearance or feel when palpated.
- Avoid areas where the vein crosses over joints.

If the IV treatment is for a life-threatening illness or injury, choice is often limited to the areas that remain open during hypoperfusion. Otherwise, limit IV access to the more distal areas of the extremities. An important concept to remember is *Choose distally, work medially*— that is, first select areas that are as distal as possible. If the distal site

> **R**emember:
>
> *Choose distally, work medially—* select distal sites when first attempting to start an IV.

ruptures, or **blows,** you can move up the extremity to the next appropriate site. Because the failed **cannulation** creates a possibility of leakage into the surrounding tissues, any fluid introduced immediately below an open wound has the potential to enter the tissue and possibly cause damage.

Large protruding arm veins can be deceiving in terms of their ease of cannulation. Often these bulging veins can "roll and blow"—that is, they will move from side to side during cannulation, causing you to miss the vein. A remedy is to apply **manual traction** to the vein to lock it into position. Traction techniques differ depending on the location chosen for cannulation. Hold hand veins in place by pulling the skin over the vein taut with the thumb of your free hand as you flex the patient's hand. Stabilize wrist veins by flexing the wrist and pulling the skin taut over the vein. Applying lateral traction to the vein with your free hand can stabilize veins in the forearm and **antecubital** areas.

The patient's opinion should also be considered when selecting an IV site, because he or she may know an IV location that has worked in the past. Avoid attempts to insert an IV in an extremity if it shows signs of trauma, injury, or infection; if it has an arteriovenous shunt for renal dialysis, or if it is on the same side as a mastectomy. Also pay careful attention to areas of the vein that have **track marks,** because this is usually a sign of **sclerosis** caused by frequent cannulation or puncture of the vein.

Some protocols allow cannulation of leg veins for IV starts. Caution must be used when cannulating these areas, because they can place the patient at greater risk of **venous thrombosis** and **pulmonary embolus.**

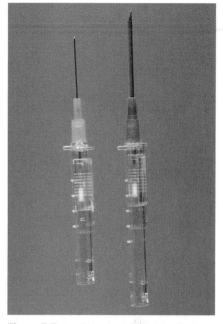

Figure 7-5 A catheter is a hollow tube that is inserted into a vein in order to keep the vein open, allowing a passageway into the vein.

Choosing a Catheter

A **catheter** is a hollow, laser-sharpened needle inside a hollow plastic tube inserted into a vein to keep the vein open (**Figure 7-5**). The most common types of catheters found in the prehospital setting are **butterfly catheters** and **over-the-needle catheters** (**Figure 7-6**). Catheter selection should reflect the need for the IV, the age of the patient, and the location for the IV.

Catheters are sized by their diameter and referred to by the **gauge** of the catheter. The larger the diameter of the catheter, the smaller the gauge. Thus, a 14-gauge catheter has a greater diameter than a 22-gauge catheter. The larger the diameter, the more fluid can be delivered through the catheter (see **Table 7-1**).

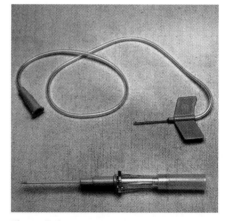

Figure 7-6 A butterfly catheter (top) and an over-the-needle catheter (bottom).

Table 7-1: Catheter Sizes and Corresponding Flow Rates		
Gauge of Catheter	Flow per Minute, mL	Flow per Hour, L
14	161	9.67
16	124	7.45
18	80	4.81

Table 7-2: Advantages and Disadvantages of Butterfly Catheters	
Advantages	**Disadvantages**
Easiest **venipuncture** device to insert	May easily cause **infiltration**
Ideal for scalp veins of children and small difficult veins in geriatric patients needing only IV access	Possible blood cell damage when drawing blood through the butterfly catheter
Small, short needles	Small-gauged needles limit fluid flow or blood draws

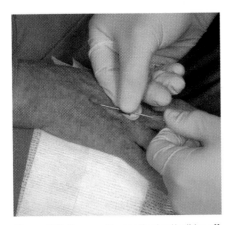

Figure 7-7 The over-the-needle sheath slides off the needle during cannulation and remains inside the vein to keep the vein open.

contaminated stick
The puncturing of an emergency care provider's skin with a catheter that was used on a patient.

Select the largest-diameter catheter that will fit the vein you have chosen or that will be the most appropriate and comfortable for the patient. A good rule of thumb to follow is: *The more distal the IV site, the smaller the catheter.* An 18-gauge catheter is usually a good size for adult patients who do not need fluid replacement. Metacarpal veins of the hand accommodate 18- to 20-gauge catheters; antecubital veins of the upper arm can accommodate larger 16- to 14-gauge catheters.

Butterfly catheters derive their name from the plastic tabs attached to the sides of the needle. These allow for a stable anchoring platform. **Table 7-2** lists the advantages and disadvantages of using butterfly catheters.

Over-the-needle catheters can be used for all adults and most children for long-term therapy (**Figure 7-7**). The plastic catheter allows for greater patient movement and often does not require immobilizing the entire limb. Over-the-needle catheters come in different gauges as well as in different lengths. The most common lengths are 2¼ inches and 1¼ inches. The shorter the catheter, the more fluid can flow through it.

In recent years, an attempt has been made to create over-the-needle catheters that minimize the risk of a contaminated stick. A **contaminated stick** occurs when the EMT punctures his or her skin with the same catheter that was used to cannulate the vein of a patient. Newer over-the-needle catheters use several different methods to protect the EMT from the possibility of a contaminated stick. One of the more common methods is automatic needle retraction after insertion, usually accomplished with a locking slide mechanism or a spring-loaded slide mechanism. As with the butterfly catheter, there are advantages and disadvantages with the over-the-needle catheters (see **Table 7-3**).

The larger a catheter's diameter, the smaller its gauge.

Table 7-3: Advantages and Disadvantages of Over-the-Needle Catheters	
Advantages	**Disadvantages**
Less likely to puncture a vein than the butterfly catheter	Risk of resticking the rescuer with contaminated needle
More comfortable once in position	More difficult to insert than other devices
Radiopaque for easy identification during x-ray	Possibility of **catheter shear**
Prevents **air embolus** during insertion	

Occasionally, cannulation of an artery occurs. Cannulation of an artery is easily recognized because bright red blood is quickly seen in the IV tubing and the IV bag because of the high pressure that exists in the arteries (**Figure 7-8**). If cannulation of an artery occurs, you must stop the IV, remove the catheter, and apply constant pressure to the site for at least 5 minutes to ensure closure of the site.

The Four Rights

Administration of IV fluid and anything else through the IV line is considered a high risk for the patient because of the possible complications that may develop. Always double-check yourself to ensure accuracy and patient safety. Carpenters have a saying: "Measure twice and cut once." This is sound advice! A pneumonic called the *four rights* is used in the medical community as a double-check:

- Do I have the *right patient?*
- Do I have the *right solution?*
- Do I have the *right drug?* (At this point, the only choice may be D_{50}.)
- Do I have the *right route?*

Inserting the IV Catheter

Each EMT has a unique technique to insert an IV, and it is important for you to observe many different techniques to determine what works best for you. The following considerations, however, are common with any technique:

- Keep the beveled side of the catheter up when inserting the needle in a vein (**Figure 7-9**).
- Maintain adequate traction on the vein during cannulation.

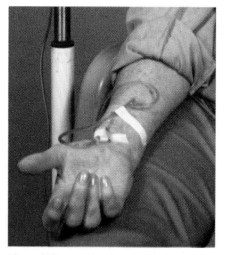

Figure 7-8 A cannulated artery can be recognized by the bright red blood quickly seen through the IV tubing due to the pressure that exists in the arteries.

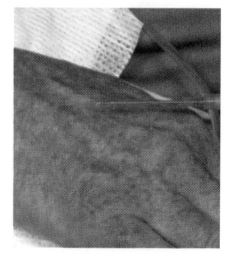

Figure 7-9 Keep the beveled side of the catheter up when inserting the needle in a vein.

Apply a constricting band above the site you have chosen for the insertion to allow blood to fill the veins. A constricting band is used to help create additional vascular pressure to engorge the veins with blood below the constricting band. Constricting bands should be snug enough to significantly diminish venous flow but should not hamper arterial flow. The constricting band should be left in place only long enough to complete the IV insertion, blood draws, and line attachment. *Do not leave the constricting band applied while you assemble IV equipment.*

Constricting bands can be difficult to manage, especially if you are wearing gloves. You should develop a technique that will allow you to release the constricting band with a small tug on one end. Constricting bands can be made of any available material, such as:

- **Penrose drains**
- Gloves
- Blood pressure cuffs
- Surgical hose

Once you have selected an insertion site, prep it with an alcohol or iodine swab. Apply gentle downward or lateral traction on the vein with your free hand while holding the catheter, bevel side up, in your dominant hand. Take care as you apply traction to avoid collapsing the vein. Begin by establishing an insertion angle of about 45°. Advance the catheter through the skin until the vein is pierced (there may or may not be a flash of blood in the catheter **flash chamber**); then immediately drop the angle down to about 15° and advance the catheter a few more centimeters to ensure the catheter sheath is in the vein. Slide the sheath off the needle and into the vein; do not advance the needle too far because it can lacerate the vein. After the catheter is fully advanced, **tamponade** off the vein just proximal to the end of the indwelling catheter, remove the needle, and dispose of it in a sharps container.

Drawing Blood

Drawing blood, while preferable, is not always possible. Often a patient is so compromised that it is impossible to obtain blood draws. If you are having difficulty drawing blood, stop and finish the IV. *Do not allow the constricting band to remain tied too long* around the patient's arm because this will allow waste products to build up in the blood and will skew lab results. Attach the **Vacutainer** to the hub of the catheter

When performing a blood draw, do not shake the red-topped tube after the blood has clotted; this will destroy the sample.

sheath and release the hand holding pressure because you now have a sealed system. Grasp the Vacutainer in one hand to stabilize it while you insert the tubes for the blood draws. If you don't have a Vacutainer setup, you can draw blood from the IV site through a 15- to 20-mL syringe. It is important to remember that for the tubes to be viable for testing, they need to be at least three quarters full. Follow local protocols for the types of blood tubes to draw. The tube tops usually come in red, blue, green, and lavender. You can use the following mnemonic to help remember the order for filling the tubes:

- *Red* – red top

- *Blood* – blue top

- *Gives* – green top

- *Life* – lavender top

Fill the red-topped tube first because it contains no additives and is intended to clot if blood typing is needed. The blue-topped tube should be filled next. It contains the preservative EDT and is used to help determine a patient's prothrombin time (PT) and partial pro-thrombin time (PPT). These values are used to calculate the patient's blood clotting time. The green-topped tube is filled with heparin to prevent clotting and is used to evaluate the patient's electrolyte and glucose levels. Lavender-topped tubes are filled with sodium citrate and are often used for a CBC (complete blood count) panel, including hematocrit levels.

Once the blood tubes are filled, gently turn them back and forth several times to mix the **anticoagulant** and blood evenly. *Note:* The exception is the red-topped tube, which is intended to separate the serum from the other blood components. There is no need to invert this tube because there is no additive to mix and the blood clots fairly quickly. Avoid shaking this tube after the blood has clotted, as this will destroy the sample.

Label all the tubes with patient's name, the date, the time, and your name as soon as possible to avoid mixing tubes with those of another patient.

Securing the Line

Once the catheter is in position and the contents of the IV bag are flowing properly, the site must be secured. Tape the area so that the catheter and tubing are securely anchored in case of a sudden pull on the line (**Figure 7-10**). You should tear the tape before you start the IV, because you will need one hand to stabilize the site while you tape the IV. Double back the tubing to create a loop that will act as a shock absorber if the line gets pulled accidentally. If you are required to apply an **opsite** over the catheter site, use the tape to secure the site. Avoid any circumferential taping around any extremity, because circumferential taping can act like a constricting band and stop circulation.

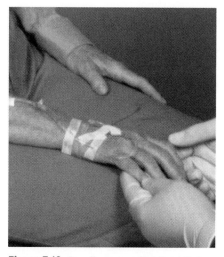

Figure 7-10 Tape the area so that the catheter and tubing are securely anchored.

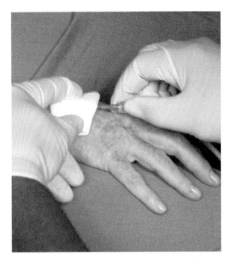

Figure 7-11 When removing a catheter and IV line, pull gently and apply pressure to control bleeding.

Discontinuing the IV Line

To discontinue the IV line, shut off the flow from the IV with the roller clamp. Gently peel the tape back *toward* the IV site. As you get closer to the site and the catheter, stabilize the catheter while you loosen all the remaining tape holding the catheter in place. Do not remove the IV tubing from the hub of the catheter. Fold a 4-inch × 4-inch piece of gauze and place it over the site, holding it down while you pull back on the hub of the catheter. Gently pull the catheter and the IV line from the patient's vein while applying pressure to control bleeding (**Figure 7-11**).

Calculations

Drug dosages and flow rate calculations are an area of confusion for most prehospital personnel, yet they are skills you will need to perform frequently, both in the field and at skill stations. Practicing the following equations is the only way to instill confidence in your abilities.

Dimensional Analysis

One of the easiest ways to figure out **drip rates,** dose calculations, weight-based calculations, and drug concentration equations is to use **dimensional analysis.** Dimensional analysis uses the same simple conversions as equations, and you will not need to memorize the equation! Dimensional analysis allows you to compare seemingly unrelated items by setting up a relationship (that is, a comparison between two items).

An example of a relationship could be a car and the wheels on a car. Every car rides on four wheels, so there are four wheels for every car.

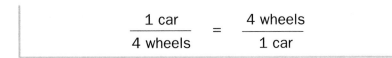

$$\frac{1 \text{ car}}{4 \text{ wheels}} = \frac{4 \text{ wheels}}{1 \text{ car}}$$

Another way to look at these comparisons is as a ratio, which is by nature a relationship. Dimensional analysis uses ratios as conversion factors.

Dosage

You can use dimensional analysis to determine dosage.

For this work you need to know:

- Dosage ordered
- Concentration of drug on hand

Example:

- Order given is for 10 mg furosemide (Lasix) IV push.

- Concentration of drug on hand is 40 mg/4 mL.

Set up the equation:

$$? \text{ mL} = \frac{4 \text{ mL}}{40 \text{ mg}} \times \frac{10 \text{ mg}}{1}$$

Be sure that you have the same terms on either side of the equal sign.

Cancel out what you can:

$$? \text{ mL} = \frac{4 \text{ mL}}{40 \; \cancel{\text{mg}}} \times \frac{10 \; \cancel{\text{mg}}}{1}$$

Reduce the fractions:

$$? \text{ mL} = \frac{4 \text{ mL}}{40} \times \frac{10}{1}$$

$$= \frac{4 \text{ mL}}{\cancel{40}} \times \frac{\cancel{10}}{1}$$

$$= \frac{\cancel{4} \text{ mL}}{\cancel{4}} \times \frac{1}{1}$$

$$= 1 \text{ mL}$$

The answer is 1 mL of furosemide (Lasix).

Drip Rates

Use dimensional analysis to solve for drip rates.

For this work you need to know:

- Which administration set to use

- Length of time for the infusion

- Amount to flow

You may need the conversion factor of 1 hr = 60 min.

Example:

- Order given is for 250 mL normal saline (NS) over 90 minutes.

- Administration set = macrodrip (10 gtt/mL).

Determine how many drops per minute should be given.

Set up the equation:

$$\frac{?\ \text{gtt}}{\text{min}} = \frac{10\ \text{gtt}}{1\ \text{mL}} \times \frac{250\ \text{mL}}{90\ \text{min}}$$

Cancel out what you can and reduce the fractions:

$$\frac{?\ \text{gtt}}{\text{min}} = \frac{\cancel{10}\ \text{gtt}}{1\ \cancel{\text{mL}}} \times \frac{250\ \cancel{\text{mL}}}{\cancel{90}\ \text{min}}$$

$$= \frac{1\ \text{gtt}}{1} \times \frac{250}{9\ \text{min}}$$

Multiply and divide:

$$= \frac{250\ \text{gtt}}{9\ \text{min}} = \frac{27.77\ \text{gtt}}{\text{min}} = 28\ \text{gtt}$$

You will need to set the drip rate at 28 gtt/min normal saline.

Drops per Minute

Another useful formula to remember is a simple drip rate calculation that gives you the number of drops per minute:

$$\frac{(\text{volume in mL}) \times (\text{drip set})}{(\text{time in minutes})} = \frac{\text{gtt}}{\text{min}}$$

Weight-Based Dosage

You may be asked to calculate the amount of a drug to give a patient based on the patient's weight. This type of problem involves two issues:

- How much drug to give
- The amount of drug to give per kilogram

Use dimensional analysis to solve for weight-based equations.

For this work you need to know:

- Patient's weight
- Amount of drug to administer

Note: You may need the conversion factor 1 kg = 2.2 lb

Example:

- Order given for 0.5 mg/kg of D_{50}
- Patient's weight = 220 lb

Determine how many milligrams need to be given.

Set up the equation:

$$? \text{ mg} = \frac{0.5 \text{ mg}}{\text{kg}} \times \frac{1.0 \text{ kg}}{2.2 \text{ lb}} \times \frac{220 \text{ lb}}{1}$$

Cancel out what you can and reduce the fractions:

$$? \text{ mg} = \frac{0.5 \text{ mg}}{\cancel{\text{kg}}} \times \frac{1.0 \cancel{\text{kg}}}{\cancel{2.2 \text{ lb}}} \times \frac{\cancel{220 \text{ lb}}}{1}$$

Multiply and divide:

$$? \text{ mg} = \frac{0.5 \text{ mg}}{1} \times \frac{1.0}{1} \times \frac{100}{1}$$

$$= 50 \text{ mg}$$

The answer is 50 mg of D_{50}.

Now, how many amp of D_{50} would be needed?

$$? \text{ amp} = \frac{1 \text{ amp}}{\cancel{50 \text{ mg}}} \times \frac{\cancel{50 \text{ mg}}}{1}$$

$$= 1.0 \text{ amp}$$

The answer is 1 amp of D_{50}.

Alternative IV Sites and Techniques

Some additional IV sites and techniques available to prehospital providers require training beyond the scope of this course. However, because you may need to assist in these types of IV administration, you can benefit from understanding how they work.

- **Saline locks (buff caps)** are a way to maintain an active IV site without having to run fluids through the vein. These access devices are used primarily for patients who do not need additional fluids but may need rapid medication delivery. Saline locks are access ports commonly used with patients who have disorders such as congestive heart failure (CHF) or pulmonary edema. A saline lock is attached to the end of an IV catheter and filled with approximately 2 mL of normal saline to keep blood from clotting at the end of the catheter (**Figure 7-12**). Because this is a sealed-access site, the saline remains in the port without entering the vein, thus preventing clotting.

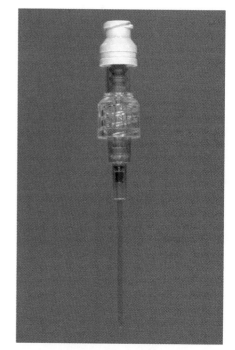

Figure 7-12 A saline lock is attached to the end of an IV catheter and fitted with approximately 2 mL of normal saline in order to keep blood from clotting at the end of the catheter.

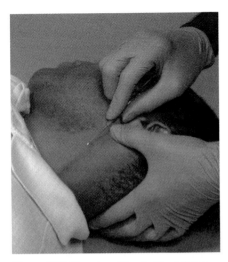

Figure 7-13 The external jugular IV requires a very specific insertion site midway between the angle of the jaw and the midclavicular line with the catheter pointed toward the shoulder of the same side as the puncture.

- **Intraosseous IVs (IOs)** are used for emergency venous access in pediatric patients as defined by protocol when immediate IV access is difficult or impossible. Often these children are experiencing a life-threatening situation such as cardiac arrest, status epilepticus, or progressive shock. IOs are established in the **proximal tibial plateau** with a rigid boring IV catheter, commonly known as a **Jamshedi needle.** This double needle, consisting of a solid boring needle inside a sharpened hollow needle, is pushed into the bone with a screwing, twisting action. Once the needle pops through the bone, the solid needle is removed, leaving the hollow steel needle in place. The IV tubing is attached to this catheter. Anything that flows through a normal IV can be infused through an IO line. Intraosseous IVs require full and careful immobilization because they rest at a 90° angle to the bone and are easily dislodged.

- **External jugular IVs** provide venous access through the external jugular veins of the neck. These are the same veins used to assess jugular vein distention (JVD). The vein is tamponaded by placing a finger on the vein above the clavicle, causing the vein to fill. The catheter is inserted into the vein in the same manner as a normal IV, except the insertion point is very specific. The catheter is inserted midway between the angle of the jaw and the mid-clavicular line, with the catheter pointed toward the shoulder on the same side as the puncture site (**Figure 7-13**). These punctures are difficult because these veins are surrounded by a very tough fibrous sheath that makes access difficult.

These techniques require more advanced training than this class will provide. Understanding their application and use is important because you may need to assist on these procedures.

Possible Complications of IV Therapy

Peripheral IV insertion carries associated risks. The problems associated with IVs can be categorized as either local or systemic reactions. **Local reactions** include problems like infiltration and phlebitis. **Systemic complications** include allergic reactions and circulatory overload.

Local IV Site Reactions

Most local reactions require that you discontinue the IV, reestablish the IV in the opposite extremity, and document the event. Some examples of local reactions include:

- Infiltration
- Phlebitis
- Occlusion
- Vein irritation
- Hematoma
- Nerve, tendon, or ligament damage

Infiltration

<u>Infiltration</u> is the escape of fluid into the surrounding tissue. This escape of fluid causes a localized area of edema. Some of the more common reasons for infiltration include the following:

- The IV has passed completely through the vein and out the other side.
- The patient is moving excessively.
- The tape used to secure the area has become loose or dislodged.
- The catheter was started at too shallow an angle and has only entered the **fascia** surrounding the vein (this is more common with IVs in larger veins, such as those in the upper arm and neck).

Some of the associated signs and symptoms of infiltration include the following:

- Edema at the catheter site
- Continued IV flow after occlusion of the vein above the insertion point
- Patient complaint of tightness and pain around the IV site

To correct the infiltration, discontinue the IV and reestablish it in the opposite extremity, or at a more proximal location on the same extremity. Apply direct pressure over the swollen area to reduce further swelling or bleeding into the tissue. Avoid wrapping tape around the extremity for direct pressure because this could create a constricting band.

Phlebitis

Phlebitis is inflammation of the vein. Phlebitis is not usually seen with the emergency prehospital patient, although you may encounter it in emergency drug abuse patients when you attempt to establish an IV. Nowadays, hospital outpatient treatment or home health care often allows the patient to receive IV therapy at home, which can also lead to phlebitis. Often phlebitis is associated with fever, tenderness, and red streaking up the associated vein. Hardening of the vein can occur if **perforation** of the vein is from repeated puncture, as seen with drug abuse. Some of the more common causes for phlebitis include localized irritation and infection from nonsterile equipment, prolonged IV therapy, or irritating IV solutions. If the phlebitis is associated with the IV you have started, discontinue the IV and reestablish it in another location, using new equipment.

Occlusion

<u>Occlusion</u> is the physical blockage of a vein or catheter. If the flow rate is not sufficient to keep fluid moving out of the catheter tip and if blood enters the catheter, a clot may form and occlude the flow. The first sign of a possible occlusion is a decreasing drip rate or the presence of blood in the IV tubing. Occlusion can be caused by a positional IV site—that is, fluid flows at different rates depending on the position of the catheter within the vein. Close proximity to a valve is often the reason for positional IVs. Other causes can be related to patient movement that allows the line to become physically blocked from either resting on the line or crossing arms. Occlusion may also develop if the IV bag nears empty and the blood pressure overcomes the flow and backs up in the line.

Use the steps shown in **Box 7-4** to determine whether the IV should be reestablished.

<u>infiltration</u>
The escape of fluid into the surrounding tissue.

<u>occlusion</u>
The physical blockage of a vein or catheter.

Box 7-4: **Determining if an IV is Viable**

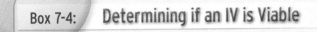

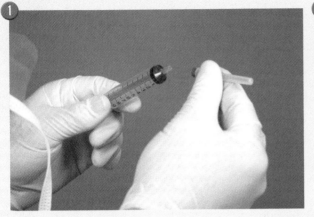

1 Select and assemble a sterile 10-mL syringe and large-gauge needle.

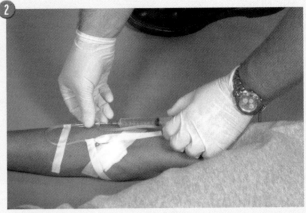

2 Select an injection port close to the IV site and wipe it with an alcohol wipe.

Depress the plunger of the syringe and insert the syringe into the port.

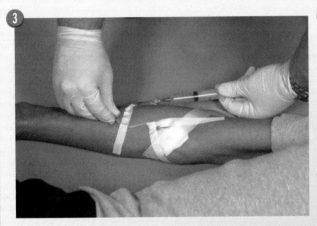

3 Pinch the line between the IV site and the port and pull back on the plunger to draw clean IV fluid from the bag.

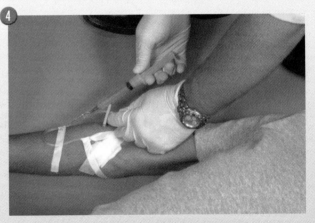

4 Once the syringe is full, leave it in place and switch your hand from the tubing between the port and the IV site to between the port and the IV bag, then pinch the line.

Now you have a full syringe of clean IV fluid and a way to add pressure to the line. Gently apply pressure to the plunger to disrupt the occlusion and reestablish flow.

If flow is reestablished, ensure that the line is free and the rate is sufficient.

If the occlusion does not dislodge, discontinue the IV and reestablish it either in the opposite extremity or at a proximal location on the same extremity.

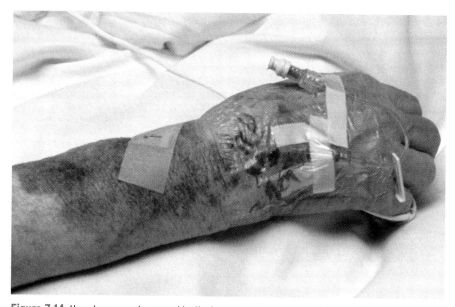

Figure 7-14 Hematomas can be caused by the improper removal of a catheter, resulting in the pooling of blood around the IV site, leading to tenderness and pain.

Vein Irritation

Occasionally, a patient will experience vein irritation in reaction to the fluid used for an IV. Patients who have this problem often complain immediately that the solution is bothering them. It may tingle, sting, or itch. Note these complaints and observe the patient closely in case he or she develops a more serious allergic reaction to the fluid.

The cause of vein irritation is usually a too rapid infusion of an irritating solution. If redness develops at the IV site with rapidly developing phlebitis, discontinue the IV and save it for later analysis. Reestablish the IV in the other extremity with all new equipment in case there were unseen contaminates in the old equipment. Be sure to document the event and the patient's response.

Hematoma

A **hematoma** is an accumulation of blood in the tissues surrounding an IV site. Hematomas result from vein perforation or improper catheter removal which allows blood to accumulate in the surrounding tissues. Blood can be seen rapidly pooling around the IV site, leading to tenderness and pain (**Figure 7-14**). Patients with a history of vascular diseases (diabetes) or patients on certain drug therapies (such as corticosteroids) can have a predisposition to vein rupture or have tendencies to develop hematomas rapidly on IV insertion.

If a hematoma develops while you are attempting to insert a catheter, stop and apply direct pressure to help minimize bleeding. If a hematoma develops after a successful catheter insertion, evaluate the IV flow and the hematoma. If the hematoma appears to be controlled and the flow is not affected, monitor the IV site and leave the line in place. If the hematoma develops as a result of discontinuing the IV, apply direct pressure with a piece of 4-inch × 4-inch gauze to the site.

hematoma
An accumulation of blood in the tissues surrounding an IV site.

It is important to carefully document each administration of IV therapy. Include the patient's chief complaint, your observations, assessment, and treatment provided.

Nerve, Tendon, or Ligament Damage

Improper identification of anatomic structures around the IV site can lead to perforation of tendons, ligaments, or nerves. An IV site choice around joints increases the risk for perforation of these structures. Patients will experience sudden and severe shooting pain when a nerve, tendon, or ligament is perforated. Numbness in the extremity after the incident can be common. Immediately remove the catheter and select another IV site. Be sure to document the event.

Systemic Complications

Systemic complications can evolve from reactions or complications associated with IV insertion. Systemic complications usually involve other body systems and can be life threatening. If the IV line is established and patent, do not remove it, because it may be needed for treatment of the patient. Common systemic complications are:

- Allergic reactions
- Air embolus
- Catheter shear
- Circulatory overload
- Vasovagal reactions

Allergic Reactions

Often allergic reactions are minor, but true **anaphylaxis** is possible and must be treated aggressively. Allergic reactions can be related to an individual's unexpected sensitivity to an IV fluid or medication. Such a sensitivity could be an unknown condition to the patient; thus, vigilance must be maintained with any IV for a possible reaction.

Patient presentation depends on the extent of the reaction. Common signs and symptoms of an allergic reaction include:

- Itching
- Edema of face and hands
- Bronchospasm
- Wheezing
- Shortness of breath
- Urticaria
- Anaphylaxis

If an allergic reaction occurs, discontinue the IV and remove the solution. Leave the catheter in place as an emergency medication route. Notify medical control immediately and maintain an open airway. Monitor ABCs and vital signs. Document the event and keep the solution or medication for evaluation by the hospital.

Air Embolus

Healthy adults can tolerate as much as 200 mL of air introduced into the circulatory system, but patients who are already ill or injured can be affected if any air is introduced into the IV line. Properly flushing an IV line will help eliminate any potential of introducing air into a patient. IV bags are designed to collapse as they empty to help prevent this problem, but collapse does not always occur. Be sure to replace empty IV bags with full ones.

If your patient begins developing respiratory distress with unequal breath sounds, consider the possibility of an air embolus. Other associated signs and symptoms include:

- Cyanosis (even in the presence of high-flow oxygen)

- Signs and symptoms of shock

- Loss of consciousness

- Respiratory arrest

Treat a patient with a suspected air embolus by placing the patient on his or her left side with the head down to trap any air inside the right atrium or right ventricle. Be prepared to ventilate the patient if he or she experiences increasing shortness of breath. Document the event.

Catheter Shear

Catheter shear occurs when part of the catheter is pinched against the needle, and the needle slices through the catheter, creating a free-floating segment. This allows the catheter segment to travel through the circulatory system and possibly end up in the pulmonary circulation, causing a pulmonary embolus.

Treatment involves surgical removal of the sheared tip. Catheter hubs are radiopaque (that is, they will appear white in an X-ray) to aid in diagnosing this type of problem. Never rethread a catheter—dispose of the used one and use a clean one.

Patients who have experienced catheter shear present with sudden **dyspnea**, shortness of breath, and possibly diminished breath sounds. They will mimic the presentations of the air embolus patient and can be treated the same way. Such patients will need continued IV access, and you must try to obtain an IV site in the other extremity.

Circulatory Overload

An unmonitored IV bag can lead to circulatory overload. Healthy adults can handle as much as 2 to 3 extra liters of fluid without compromise. Problems occur when the patient has cardiac, pulmonary, or renal dysfunction. These types of dysfunction do not tolerate any additional demands from increased circulatory volume. The most common cause for circulatory overload in the prehospital setting is failure to readjust the drip rate after flushing an IV line immediately after insertion. Always monitor IV bags to ensure the proper drip rate.

Patient presentation includes dyspnea, JVD, and increased blood pressure. Crackles are often heard when evaluating breath sounds. Acute peripheral edema can also be an indication of circulatory overload.

To treat a patient with circulatory overload, slow the IV rate to keep the vein open and raise the patient's head to ease respiratory distress. Administer high-flow oxygen and monitor vital signs and shortness of breath. Contact medical control immediately and inform them of the developing problem, because there are drugs that can be given to reduce the circulatory volume. Document the event.

Vasovagal Reactions

Some patients have anxiety concerning needles or in response to the sight of blood. Such anxiety may cause vasculature dilation, leading to a drop in blood pressure and patient collapse. Patients can present with anxiety, diaphoresis, nausea, and **syncopal episodes.**

> **P**atients experiencing air embolus or catheter shear present with similar symptoms and can be treated by the same methods.

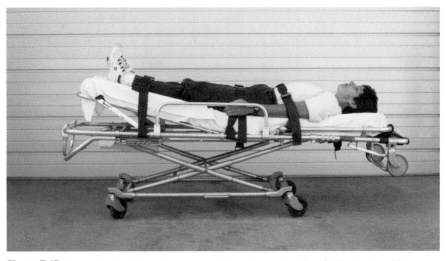

Figure 7-15 When patients collapse due to vasovagal reactions, place them in the shock position.

vasovagal reaction
Sudden hypotension and fainting associated with a traumatic or medical event.

Treatment for patients with **vasovagal reactions** centers on treating them for shock:

1. Place patient in **shock position** (**Figure 7-15**).
2. Apply high-flow oxygen.
3. Monitor vital signs.
4. Establish an IV in case fluid resuscitation is needed.

Troubleshooting

Several factors can influence the flow rate of an IV. For example, if the IV bag is not hung high enough, the flow rate will not be sufficient. It is always helpful to perform the following checks after completing IV administration. Also, if there is a flow problem, rechecking these items will help determine the problem.

- *Check your IV fluid.*
  Thick, viscous fluids such as blood products and colloid solutions infuse slowly and may be diluted to help speed delivery. Cold fluids run slower than warm fluids. If you can, warm IV fluids before administering them in cold months.

- *Check your administration set.*
  Macrodrips are used for rapid fluid delivery, whereas microdrips are designed to deliver a more controlled flow.

- *Check the height of your IV bag.*
  The IV bag must be hung high enough to overcome the patient's own blood pressure. Hang the bag as high as possible.

- *Check the type of catheter used.*
  The wider the catheter (the smaller the gauge), the more fluid can be delivered; 14 gauge is the widest, 27 gauge the narrowest.

- *Check your constricting band.*
  One of the most overlooked factors in IV flow rate is leaving the constricting band on the patient's arm after completing the IV.

Wrap Up

Chapter 7
IV Techniques and Administration

Ready for Review

Successful IV technique takes time to perfect. Several factors, from the patient's condition to the available IV equipment, influence every IV start. Mastery of IV skills comes when you understand and can overcome all the variables. Take your time when practicing IV starts and gain a solid understanding of what you are doing. This understanding will be useful when you need to perform a quick and flawless IV start in less than optimum conditions.

NOTE: *The solutions to questions 4 and 5 can be found in Appendix B, "Solutions to IV Calculations."*

Quick Quiz

Answer each question in your own words and perform the calculations.

1 Summarize the process of inserting a catheter into a vein.

_____

_____

2 Describe how you would correctly assemble the bag and blood tubing.

_____

_____

3 Calculate the drip rate for administering 500 mL of normal saline through a macrodrip set over 45 minutes.

_____

_____

4 Perform the following calculations:

a. Order: morphine sulfate (MSO_4) 2 mg IV push
On hand: 10 mg/mL morphine sulfate in prefilled syringe
How many mL would you administer?

b. Order: bretylium tosylate 5 mg/kg
On hand: bretylium tosylate 500 mg/10 mL
Patient's weight: 242 lb
How many mL would you administer?

c. Order: lactated Ringer's solution 300 mL over 30 minutes
On hand: lactated Ringer's solution 1,000 mL
Admin. set 10 gtt/mL
How many gtt/min will you administer?

d. Order: Normal saline 1,000 mL over 4 hours
On hand: Normal saline 1,000 mL
Admin. set: 15 gtt/mL
How many gtt/min will you administer?

5 The patient is receiving MSO_4 via IV infusion. The concentration of the solution is 100 mg MSO_4 in 500 mL IV fluid. It is infusing at a rate of 30 mL/hr. How many mg/hr is the patient receiving?

_____

_____

Age-Specific Considerations

Pediatric and geriatric populations warrant specific attention. What sets these populations apart are (1) physical differences specific to these populations; and (2) communication barriers that prevent these patients from expressing themselves.

Accordingly, pediatric and geriatric patients have different medical needs from the general medical population, making it sometimes necessary to use other methods of assessment and treatment. This chapter will discuss the differences in pediatric and geriatric populations and explore the implications of these differences to IV therapy.

Pediatric Patients

Children are not "little adults" and cannot be treated as such. When children are injured or ill, their condition can be worsened by their natural fear of strangers or their perception of the situation. Rushing up to an infant or a small child can have a damaging outcome. Being aware of the mental and developmental changes and landmarks common with children can aid you in treating pediatric patients.

Developmental landmarks for children can be grouped according to their age:

- *Neonates* range in age from birth to 1 month old and are completely dependent on adults for support. At this age, they tolerate separation from the parent, and most responses are purely reflexive. Common illnesses include GI disturbances and respiratory problems; congenital problems can also be a concern.

- *Infants* range in age from 1 month to 1 year. At this age, a great deal of muscle development occurs, and infants begin walking. They also begin identifying with their parents or caregivers and can experience separation anxiety. Trauma starts to become a greater concern as infants explore their environment (**Figure 8-1**).

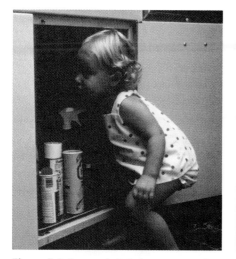

Figure 8-1 Trauma starts to become more of a concern as children explore their environment.

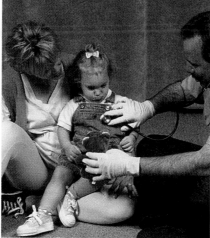

Figure 8-2 Use parents and caregivers when assessing toddlers to facilitate the process.

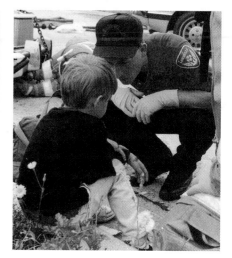

Figure 8-3 Preschoolers are distinctly aware of what is happening to them and should be told what to expect.

- *Toddlers* range in age from 1 year to 3 years. Toddlers are very aware of strangers and start to develop independence. They are often difficult to manage because they have definite opinions of what they do and do not like. Touching them, assessing them, removing their clothing, and using equipment can induce fear and apprehension. Use the help of parents or caregivers when assessing toddlers (**Figure 8-2**). Above all, remain patient.

- *Preschoolers* range in age from 3 to 6 years. They take statements literally and their imaginations can misinterpret what they do not understand, so you must take care in speaking to them. Preschoolers are distinctly aware of what is happening to them and should be told what to expect during an examination (**Figure 8-3**).

- *School-age children* range in age from 6 to 12 years. This age group tolerates separation from parents and caregivers and usually cooperates when being examined. Modesty is an issue, however.

- *Adolescents* range from age 12 to 18 years. Adolescents are experimenters who often view themselves as invincible. They will therefore push their limits by engaging in risky behaviors. At the same time, adolescents will frequently hide their experimentation from adults, including EMS personnel. They often find comfort in the company of others, either parents or friends, which may be a consideration when treating adolescents.

Parents and caregivers who overtreat or mistreat by providing medication or home remedies are another concern with pediatric patients. Parents and caregivers often make the mistake of thinking they can treat children with adult medications and adult procedures. However, medications for adults are often harmful for pediatric patients.

Children should be approached
and handled differently depending on their age.

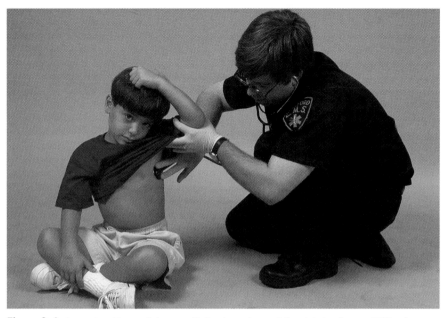

Figure 8-4 Assess breath sounds by auscultation in each armpit to minimize the possibility of hearing echoes of breath sounds from the opposite lung.

Pediatric Patient Assessment

Initial assessment of pediatric patients needs to reflect the adequacy of perfusion. Adequate pediatric perfusion is directly related to the adequacy of respiration in the lungs and the cells of the body. Assess the following three main items in pediatric patients to determine whether there is adequate perfusion:

- Appearance
- Breathing
- Circulation

Appearance refers to the child's mental status, muscle tone, and body position. Assess the mental status of the child as appropriate for his or her age group. Note the body position and muscle tone. Specifically ask caregivers if the patient's presentation is normal or if there are any changes—even slight ones. Watch parent/patient interactions. Throughout your assessment, trust your initial gut feelings.

Breathing assessment involves monitoring the chest and abdomen for adequate movement and air exchange. Assess breath sounds by **auscultation** in each armpit to minimize the possibility of hearing echoes of breath sounds from the opposite lung (**Figure 8-4**). Assessing breath sounds can be difficult with young children. Instead of using auscultation, you may need to look at the chest or abdomen for movement to evaluate adequate air exchange. Be on guard for any possible chest injury that could affect respiratory assessment and ventilation.

Adequate perfusion for pediatric patients is directly related to adequate respiration.

Circulation assessment involves evaluating the pulses (peripheral and central) and examining skin color, temperature, and capillary refill. Blood pressure (BP) is less important and less accurate for children under 3 years of age. Instead, assess the adequacy of perfusion by monitoring pulses and capillary refill (**Figure 8-5**). If it becomes necessary to obtain the blood pressure of the child, you can calculate expected values using the following formulas.

To calculate the lower limit for a child's normal systolic blood pressure, use the following equation:

$$BP = (2 \times \text{age in years}) + 70$$

To calculate the lower limit for a child's normal pulse rate, use the following equation:

$$\text{Rate} = 150 - (5 \times \text{age in years})$$

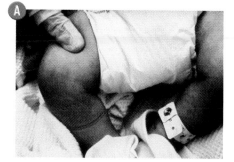

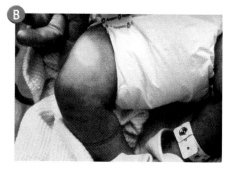

Figure 8-5 Assess the adequacy of perfusion by monitoring pulses and capillary refill.

The Pediatric Trauma Patient

Pediatric injuries are an important concern for EMTs. The latest statistics show that pediatric injuries occur more often than all other pediatric problems combined. Injuries claim the lives of over 20,000 pediatric patients every year in the United States. The American Academy of Pediatrics estimates that one in four children will be injured enough to require some form of emergency department care. **Table 8-1** lists the leading causes of pediatric injury and death in the United States.

Table 8-1: Leading Causes of Death in the United States			
1-4 years	5-9 years	10-14 years	15-24 years
① Motor vehicle traffic	Motor vehicle traffic	Motor vehicle traffic	Motor vehicle traffic
② Congenital abnormalities	Malignant neoplasms	Malignant neoplasms	Homicide
③ Drowning	Drowning	Suicide	Suicide
④ Homicide	Congenital abnormalities	Homicide	Malignant neoplasms
⑤ Malignant neoplasms	Fires/burns	Drowning	Heart disease

Source: Adapted from the CDC, National Center for Injury Prevention, Leading Causes of Death Reports, 1998.

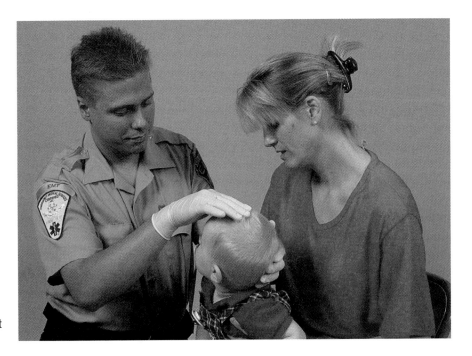

Figure 8-6 Infants with closed head injuries must be evaluated for signs and symptoms of shock.

Evaluation of pediatric trauma includes evaluation of the mechanism of injury (MOI). Higher-risk MOIs are associated with injury to the head and neck, fractures to the extremities, and **thoracoabdominal** injuries. Higher-risk MOIs include the following:

- Motor vehicle crashes (improperly restrained passenger)
- Auto versus pediatric pedestrian crashes
- Air bag injuries
- Falls (greater than three times the patient's height)
- Swimming/diving injuries
- Bicycle crashes in which the child is not wearing a helmet
- "Up and over" pediatric bicycle crashes involving handlebar injuries

Infants with closed head injuries must be evaluated for the development of shock (**Figure 8-6**). Closed head injuries in pediatric patients have a different course from closed head injuries in other age groups. Infant blood volumes and cranial vaults are large, so there is room for blood to accumulate and shock to develop before the signs of a closed head injury may be seen. **Unfused cranial plates** allow for injury transfer to underlying brain tissue and for expansion of the brain tissue once bleeding and swelling begin.

Blunt force trauma to a child's chest can cause significant damage to underlying tissues because the rib cage is extremely pliable. Pediatric ribs bend quite a bit and thus allow the energy to transfer directly to the lungs, heart, liver, and abdominal organs. These injuries can generate significant blood loss from ruptured organs without outwardly obvious signs of trauma. Mechanism of injury plays a major role in determining the extent of injuries to a pediatric patient.

Pediatric Trauma Assessment

A pediatric trauma scale has been developed for the evaluation of pediatric trauma patients, similar to the Glasgow coma scale or the modified trauma scale. Add all the category totals together for a final trauma score (see **Table 8-2**). Patients with scores of 8 or less are considered critical and need **advanced life support (ALS)** and trauma center activation.

FYI

Table 8-2: Pediatric Trauma Score

	+2	+1	-1
Weight (kg*)	Greater than 20 kg (44 lb)	10 to 20 kg (22 to 44 lb)	Less than 10 kg (22 lb)
Airway	Normal	Maintained with suctioning	Maintained with jaw thrust or adjunct
Systolic BP (or central pulse)	Greater than 90 mm Hg (Strong CP)	50 to 90 mm Hg (Weak CP)	Less than 50 mm Hg (Very weak CP)
Central nervous system (AVPU)	Awake (A, alert)	Sleepy (V or P)	Coma (U, unresponsive)
Open wound	None	Minor (Small lacerations)	Major (Penetrating wounds to chest or abdomen)
Skeletal trauma	None	Closed (Arm or leg injury with swelling)	Open/multiple (Injuries or open wound near fracture)

Source: Adapted from J. J. Tepas III, D. L. Mollitt, and J. L. Talbert, "The Pediatric Trauma Score as a Predictor of Injury Severity in the Injured Child," *Journal of Pediatric Surgery 24* (1987): 14-18.

* 1 kilogram = 2.2 pounds

The Pediatric Shock Patient

Pediatric patients can suffer the same types of shock as adults (see Chapter 5, "Causes and Treatment of Shock"), although there are some differences, which are addressed below.

Respiratory failure and the development of shock are the two most significant life threats to pediatric trauma patients. Development of shock in pediatric patients is much more serious than in adults. The two main causes of shock in children are:

- Trauma resulting in internal or external bleeding
- Repeated vomiting or diarrhea, especially if there is no fluid intake

Table 8-3: Pediatric Shock Assessment

Assessment	Normal	Early	Late
Pulse rate	Normal	Fast	Very fast or slow
Central pulse	Normal	Normal	Weak
Peripheral pulse	Normal	Weak	Absent
Skin color (extremities)	Normal	Cyanotic	Systemic cyanosis
Skin temperature	Normal	Cool	Cool/clammy
Capillary refill	2 to 3 seconds	Delayed (3 to 5 seconds)	Very delayed (More than 5 seconds)
*Blood pressure	Normal	Normal	Low

Source: Adapted from the Center for Pediatric Emergency Medicine, "Circulatory Assessment Findings for Pediatric Shock," *Teaching Resource for Instructors in Prehospital Pediatrics*, CD Version 2.0, 1998.

*In children 3 years of age or younger, strong central pulse is a good indication of adequate blood pressure. Blood pressure readings are less accurate for children under 3 years of age.

Any pediatric patient with significant injury or continued fluid losses from vomiting and diarrhea should be assessed carefully for shock. When assessing for respiratory failure and shock (see **Table 8-3**), follow the ABCs: direct your attention toward airway maintenance first, then to breathing and circulation.

Pediatric Septic Shock

Infants and small children are frequently affected by septic shock. Illnesses often go undetected for longer periods of time in children because they do not always verbalize that they are ill.

Signs and symptoms of pediatric septic shock include:

- Tachycardia (sometimes extreme)
- Tachypnea with rates over 60 BPM
- Decreasing LOC
- Febrile, dry skin
- Dry mucous membranes

Pediatric Hypovolemic Shock

When adults are thirsty, they get a drink. When small children or infants are thirsty, they will either ask for a drink or hope someone notices that they are thirsty. Fluid losses in small children and infants may therefore go unnoticed until significant hypovolemia is present, especially if there is an associated illness. Diarrhea and vomiting are common causes for hypovolemic shock. Fluid replacement for hypovolemic pediatric patients is 20 mL/kg of isotonic fluid.

> **B**ecause children do not always communicate that they are ill, their illnesses may go undetected longer. This puts them at a higher risk for septic shock—shock caused by a severe bacterial infection.

> **B**ecause pediatric patients may not always be properly hydrated, they are at a higher risk for hypovolemic shock. Children who have diarrhea and/or are vomiting are also at a greater risk for hypovolemic shock because they are losing fluid.

Pediatric Hemorrhagic Shock

Pediatric patients who are hemorrhaging tend to respond differently than adult patients who are hemorrhaging. Pediatric patients compensate and may not show outward signs or symptoms of shock until there is 40% or more blood loss. At that point, their blood pressure "crashes." Pediatric blood pressure is maintained through cardiac output. There are few compensatory mechanisms in place for very young patients. Hearts will pump until they bleed out. Any blood loss can be life threatening.

The Pediatric Medical Patient

Pediatric patients can experience the same illnesses and exposures as adults (see Chapter 2, "Infection Control"), but pediatric patients are more prone to infection because their immune systems are not yet fully developed. A serious situation can occur if a bacterial or viral infection develops unchecked. Serious illnesses that warrant immediate attention include meningitis, fever, and poisonings.

Meningitis. Headaches, vomiting, lethargy, pain with flexion, and altered mental status must be evaluated as possible indications of meningitis, a severe bacterial infection of the membranes surrounding the brain and spinal cord. Watch for the ominous development of a **petechial rash** on the body of the child (**Figure 8-7**).

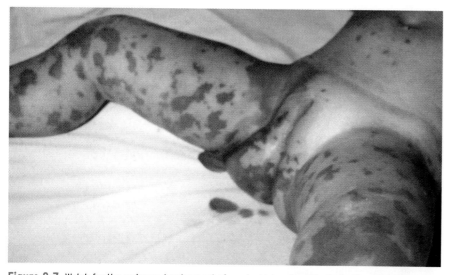

Figure 8-7 Watch for the ominous development of a petechial rash on the body of a child who may have meningitis.

Fever. Elevated temperatures are a normal immune response and are often idiopathic. Most fevers can be managed with over-the-counter medications and doctor visits. If the fever is sudden and the body temperature rises rapidly, children can suffer from febrile seizures. Fevers that do not respond to medication are a serious life threat and must be treated. Often, children with fevers are treated at home with remedies that can compound the problem. Rubbing alcohol baths can be dangerous because children can absorb the isopropyl alcohol through the skin, resulting in alcohol poisoning. Ice water baths can temporarily lower body temperature and should be used sparingly, because they can induce dangerous complications. EMTs should avoid giving pediatric patients ice water baths and should use tepid water instead. Children are at greater risk for hypothermia than adults, and prolonged submersion in ice water can produce dangerous consequences. Aspirin and pediatric fevers are a dangerous combination. A serious brain disease is possible if aspirin is used to treat fevers associated with chicken pox, influenza, or other illnesses.

Poisonings. Pediatric poisonings present another unique situation for patient management. Young pediatric patients are at a higher risk for poisonings because they explore the world by placing things in their mouths.

The most common forms of pediatric poisonings result from ingestion, especially from household items such as:

- Cleaning agents
- Plants
- Cosmetics
- Tobacco from unsmoked cigarettes

Poisonings from ingestion of medications are also common. Any medication can result in poisoning, including those that seem benign, such as aspirin and acetaminophen. According to toxicology research, an oral dose of acetaminophen greater than or equal to 150 mg/kg in a child is considered toxic. Aspirin overdoses are not as common in children but are just as dangerous. The main ingredient in aspirin is salicylate, and the most toxic form of salicylate is oil of wintergreen (methyl salicylate), often found in rubbing creams designed for muscle aches and pains. Fatal doses have been reported with ingestion of as little as 1 teaspoon.

Pediatric medications are often supplied in suspensions that mix the medications with sweet-tasting syrups to make the medication more palatable and thus more dangerous. Children often do not understand the concept of dosing and may ingest the medication out of curiosity or because it may taste good.

> **B**ecause their immune systems are not yet fully developed, children are at a higher risk for developing infections.

Potentially lethal poisonings can occur from:

- Iron supplements
- Heart and blood pressure medications
- Psychiatric drugs
- Acetaminophen (Tylenol)

Pediatric IV Therapy

The same IV solutions and equipment can be used on pediatric patients as on adults (see Chapter 7, "Intravenous Techniques and Administration"), with a few exceptions.

Catheters. If you are using over-the-needle catheters to start a pediatric IV, the 20-, 22-, 24-, or 26-gauge catheters are best for insertions (**Figure 8-8**). Butterfly catheters are ideal for pediatric patients and can be placed in the same locations as over-the-needle catheters as well as in visible scalp veins. Scalp veins are best used in younger pediatric patients. **Intraosseous** IVs can be used for difficult and emergency fluid infusions. Intraosseous IVs contain special needles that puncture through the bone tissue of the proximal **tibial plateau,** leaving the rigid catheter in place. The IV tubing is attached to the rigid catheter just as it is with flexible catheters. Stabilization is critical for these lines to maintain adequate flow. Once established, these lines work as well as peripheral lines. Starting these lines is a skill that is above the training level of this course.

> **A**ny medication can result in poisonings in pediatric patients. Although a medication may seem benign, children may take far more than the recommended dose and become poisoned as a result.

intraosseous
Into the bone; a medication delivery route.

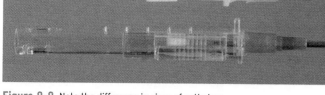

Figure 8-8 Note the difference in sizes of catheters.

> **T**he younger the pediatric patient,
>
> the more diluted the D_{50} solution needs to be.

Volutrol IV Sets. Fluid control for pediatric patients is important. Using a special type of microdrip set called a Volutrol IV allows you to fill the large drip chamber with a specific amount of fluid and administer only this amount to avoid fluid overload. The 100-mL calibrated drip chamber can be shut off from the IV bag.

IV Locations. When starting the IV, take both the child and the parent into consideration. The parent can become as stressed as the child, so take time to thoroughly explain the procedure to both the child and the parent.

The younger the pediatric patient, the fewer choices you have for IV sites. Hand veins are painful and difficult to manage in younger pediatric patients but remain the location of choice for starting peripheral IVs. Protecting the IV site after it has been established is critical and is sometimes best accomplished by immobilizing the site before cannulation with an arm board. One of the better techniques for starting pediatric IVs is to use a penlight to illuminate the veins on the back of the hand. Shine the light through the palm side of the hand to illuminate the veins on the backside of the hand. Once a suitable site is located, slightly graze the surface of the hand with your fingernail so you can find the location after you turn off the penlight. Proceed with the IV, using the mark you created as guide. Sometimes the best choice is an AC (antecubital vein) line with full arm immobilization to avoid dislodging the IV.

Scalp vein cannulation is often aesthetically unpleasant for both the child and the parents and can produce apprehension in both simply because of the location. In addition, scalp veins can be difficult to cannulate and do not allow for rapid fluid resuscitation. When securing a scalp vein, tape a paper cup over the site to avoid applying any direct pressure to the butterfly catheter. Pressure may cause the catheter to puncture the other side of the vein and let fluids escape into the tissues (extravasation).

Pediatric IV Dextrose. When administering dextrose, you must take the same precautions for both pediatric and adult patients. Before administering IV D_{50} to pediatric patients, you must dilute it into the appropriate concentration according to the patient's age:

- D_{50} can be used for pediatric patients older than 14 years of age.

- D_{25} can be used for children from 3 months to 14 years of age. Dilute $1/2$ amp of D_{50} with normal saline and deliver a 2 mL/kg IV push.

- D_{10} can be used for newborns and children up to 3 months of age. Dilute 1 mL of D_{50} in 9 mL of normal saline and deliver a 2 mL/kg IV push.

Geriatric Patients

There are an estimated 56 million senior citizens in the United States, or roughly 13% of the population. The number of senior citizens continues to increase annually, so it is safe to predict that the number of EMS patient contacts with this population will also increase. Like the pediatric population, the elderly population has its own special considerations regarding assessment and treatment.

Assessment of the Geriatric Patient

Once you have taken care of the initial ABCs, you will need to consider other issues when caring for the geriatric patient.

Legal Issues. Elderly patients are of legal age but, like other patients, they may have competency issues. It is important to establish the level of competency of an elderly patient.

Personal Issues. Routine is important and helps create a sense of security. Changes in daily routine can be very stressful for geriatric patients. In addition, elderly patients are often very independent and self-sufficient; they may fear being taken to the hospital for treatment because it means a loss of control, which can be extremely traumatic. In assisting geriatric patients, you may need to respond to some of their concerns regarding pet care, household security, and contacting friends or family.

Medications. Both prescription and over-the-counter medications can cause fragile skin and veins, excessive bleeding, poor systemic responses, and altered LOC in geriatric patients. Often, the elderly patient is under the care of several doctors, and the doctors may be unaware of the full range of treatments the elderly patient is receiving. By obtaining a full list of the patient's medications, you could be taking the first step in uncovering potential drug interactions (**Figure 8-9**).

> **C**onsider legal, personal, and medical issues when caring for a geriatric patient.

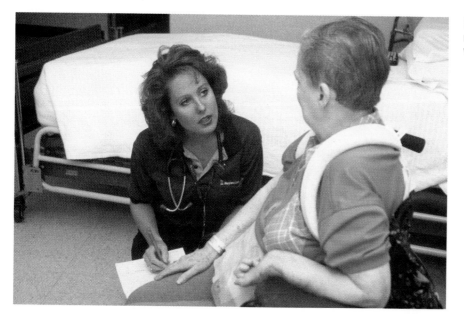

Figure 8-9 It is useful to list all of the medications the patient is taking, especially when assessing geriatric patients.

> **G**eriatric trauma patients are at a higher risk for mortality because of the medical complications of aging.

The Geriatric Trauma Patient

The mortality rate in the geriatric trauma patient is high because of the normal medical complications of aging. Reflexes are diminished, creating greater opportunity for injury. Physiologic changes in body systems (cardiovascular, musculoskeletal, respiratory, nervous, etc.) also decrease the geriatric patient's ability to react to impending injury. The normal defensive response systems begin to deteriorate, leaving the body unprotected in the event of injury. Healing processes are also compromised, making recovery difficult.

In assessing geriatric patients for trauma, you also need to address their higher tolerance for pain, which results in part from physiologic changes (for example, poor vascular circulation). Geriatric patients also have decreased cardiovascular reserves, making them extremely susceptible to compromise during any trauma event. Remaining alert for changes in patient condition and responding appropriately is very important.

Shock in the Geriatric Patient

Geriatric patients may have underlying medical conditions that are less tolerant of the possibility of shock; for example, cardiac and respiratory diseases can exacerbate problems. Often elderly patients are being treated for these conditions with medications that prevent the systemic defense mechanisms from compensating for shock. For example, to control hypertension, some medications inhibit the release of epinephrine. Lack of epinephrine can be a huge detriment to a patient with shock, because epinephrine is a major factor in the response to shock.

Geriatric Septic Shock. Elderly patients can have compromised immune systems and sedentary lifestyles, which can lead to systemic infections. Minor infections can potentially lead to septic presentations.

Geriatric Hypovolemic Shock Elderly patients may have poor nutritional or lifestyle habits that can lead to the following signs and symptoms of dehydration:

- **Skin tenting**, or poor skin turgor
- Dry mucous membranes
- Pale conjunctiva
- Decreased LOC

> **G**eriatric patients are at a greater risk for shock because of common geriatric medical conditions (such as cardiac and respiratory diseases) and medications that could interfere with the body's compensating mechanisms in response to shock.

Chronic dehydration leaves the elderly patient at an even greater risk for developing of hypovolemic shock. The simple act of sweating as a normal response to high surrounding temperatures can potentially result in hypovolemic shock. IV fluid therapy can quickly alleviate the complications of hypovolemia, but the extra fluid can be dangerous for some elderly patients if it is delivered too quickly.

Geriatric Hemorrhagic Shock.   Hemorrhagic shock in the elderly can be very serious. To control blood pressure, elderly patients may be taking medications that suppress the systemic nervous system. Suppressing this response prevents the body from compensating with its normal protective mechanisms—tachycardia and vasoconstriction. Be very careful when assessing elderly patients who are bleeding, because they may not show any changes in vital signs until they reach fatal, irreversible shock from severe blood loss.

> **E**lderly patients who are bleeding are at an increased risk for hemorrhagic shock because they may be taking medication that suppresses the systemic nervous system.

The Geriatric Medical Patient

Geriatric patients often experience multiple problems simultaneously. When you encounter a patient with a medical complaint, be sure to determine if there are any other medical problems or histories that could help explain his or her current condition (**Figure 8-10**). Ask patients specific questions about other problems relating to organ systems, such as "Do you have any heart, liver, or lung problems?" or "Do you have a history of chronic obstructive pulmonary disease (COPD), diabetes, or cardiac problems?" Often, you will find that there are other underlying conditions that can either contribute to, or be affected by, the patient's current complaints. To avoid confusing or agitating the patient, allow some time so the patient can think and respond to your questions.

Medications can play a big role in the patient's condition or presentation. They can also give clues to the extent of the patient's medical history. Locate all prescribed and over-the-counter medications, do a pill inventory to ensure the patient is taking the proper doses, and note any discrepancies in pill counts. Document all the names of the different medications as well as any doctors' names you find.

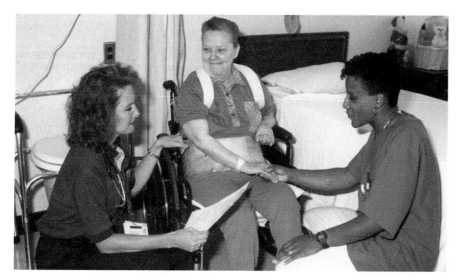

Figure 8-10 When you encounter a patient with a medical complaint, be sure to determine if there are any other medical problems or histories that could help explain the patient's current condition.

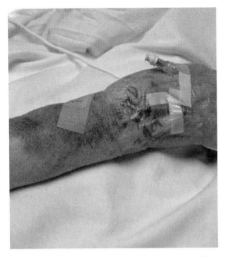

Figure 8-11 Often, simply puncturing a geriatric patient's vein will cause a massive hematoma.

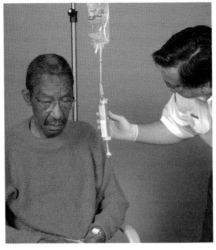

Figure 8-12 If necessary, use the Volutrol IV set to prevent fluid overload.

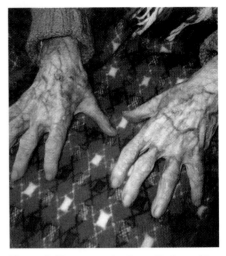

Figure 8-13 When looking for an IV site, avoid small spidery veins and varicose veins.

IV Therapy in the Geriatric Patient

Smaller catheters may be preferable with the elderly patient unless rapid fluid replacement is needed. Some medications commonly used by the elderly patient have the tendency to create fragile skin and veins. Often, simply puncturing the vein will cause a massive hematoma (**Figure 8-11**). The use of tape can lead to skin damage, so be careful when establishing IVs on the elderly.

Catheters. Try using the smaller catheters (such as 20-, 22-, or 24-gauge), because they may be more comfortable for the patient and can reduce the risk of extravasation. If fluid resuscitation is necessary, choose an appropriately sized catheter.

IV Sets. Be careful when using macrodrips, because they can allow rapid infusion of fluids, which may lead to edema if they are not monitored closely. With both geriatric and pediatric patients, fluid overloading is a real possibility. If necessary, use the Volutrol IV set to prevent fluid overloads (**Figure 8-12**).

Locations. In choosing an IV site, you should consider the possibility of poor vein elasticity. One of the consequences of aging is the loss of elasticity in the body tissues. Veins become sclerosed, making them brittle. Certain medications, like prednisone, can also affect the structure of the vein, making the veins of geriatric patients even more fragile and easily ruptured. Avoid small **spidery veins** that weave back and forth (**Figure 8-13**), because they may rupture easily. Be careful of **varicose veins;** although they often appear to be ideal choices for IV starts, they are almost completely closed off and allow very little circulation.

Because geriatric patients have more delicate skin,

use extra care when administering IVs and when applying tape to stabilize IVs.

Wrap Up

**Chapter 8
Age-Specific Considerations**

Ready for Review

Administering IVs to pediatric and geriatric patients requires special care. Both populations are at a higher risk for certain medical conditions that can affect both the patient's need for IV therapy and the effectiveness of the therapy. By understanding the risks and concerns of these populations, you will be better equipped to properly administer IV therapy. Finally, in any medical situation involving pediatric or geriatric patients, remember to be sensitive to the patient's personal issues.

Quick Quiz

Answer each question below in your own words.

1. Discuss the problem associated with blunt chest trauma in children.

2. Discuss the fluid replacement rule for pediatric patients.

3. What is one type of IV set used to regulate fluid delivery in pediatric patients?

4. How can prescription drugs affect an elderly patient who is hemorrhaging?

5. Discuss the possible problems associated with inserting IVs and securing the IV lines in elderly patients.

Appendix 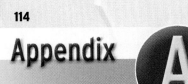 A

Review Questions: Major Concepts

1. Discuss the importance of BSI. List infectious diseases and measures that can be taken to avoid exposure. (Chapter 2: Infection Control)

2. What are the differences between hypoglycemia and diabetic ketoacidosis? Make a list differentiating between the signs and symptoms of each. (Chapter 6: Altered Level of Consciousness)

3. Discuss the differences between hypovolemic shock, hemorrhagic shock, neurogenic shock, anaphylactic shock, and distributive shock. (Chapter 5: Causes and Treatment of Shock)

4. List and describe the legal issues for the EMT. (Chapter 1: Introduction to IV Therapy: Roles, Responsibilities, and Legal Issues)

5. Identify the effects of common complications associated with IV insertion. (Chapter 7: IV Techniques and Administration)

6. What is a buffer? What is its function in the body? (Chapter 4: Principles of Fluid Balance)

7. Identify the various types of IV solutions based on their tonicity. What effect does each type have on surrounding fluid compartments? (Chapter 4: Principles of Fluid Balance)

8. Explain how each compartment of the buffering system works. List the end products that are produced by each compartment. (Chapter 4: Principles of Fluid Balance)

9. List the indications and contraindications for the use of PASG. Give reasons for each indication and contraindication. (Chapter 5: Causes and Treatment of Shock)

10. Give the indications for using D_{50}. (Chapter 6: Altered Level of Consciousness)

11. What are the different ways in which the cell can move water and substrates in and out of the cell through the cell wall? Give the name for each of these processes and explain how each works. (Chapter 3: Basic Cell Physiology)

12. Explain how to choose an IV site. Also, explain how you assess whether or not you have correctly entered the vein. (Chapter 7: Intravenous Techniques and Administration)

13. Indicate the best catheter sizes and sites for pediatric and geriatric patients. (Chapter 8: Age-Specific Considerations)

14. What are the volumes of the different fluid compartments in the body? (Chapter 3: Basic Cell Physiology)

15. List the different electrolytes in the body. (Chapter 3: Basic Cell Physiology)

16. Identify different IV sets and their properties. (Chapter 7: Intravenous Techniques and Administration)

Appendix 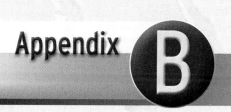 B

Solutions to IV Calculations

4. a. Ordered: 2 mg morphine sulfate (MSO$_4$)
On hand: 10 mg/mL morphine sulfate in prefilled syringe

$$?mL \quad = \quad \frac{1\ mL}{10\ mg} \quad x \quad \frac{2\ mg}{1} \quad = \quad \frac{1\ mL}{10\ \cancel{mg}} \quad x \quad \frac{2\ \cancel{mg}}{1}$$

$$= \quad \frac{2\ mL}{10}$$

$$= \quad 0.2\ mL$$

b. Ordered: bretylium tosylate 5 mg/kg
On hand: bretylium tosylate 500 mg/10 mL prefilled syringe
Patient's weight: 242 lb

$$?mL \quad = \quad \frac{10\ mL}{500\ mg} \quad x \quad \frac{5\ mL}{kg} \quad x \quad \frac{1\ kg}{2.2\ lb} \quad x \quad \frac{242\ lb}{1}$$

$$= \quad \frac{10\ mL}{500\ \cancel{mg}} \quad x \quad \frac{5\ \cancel{mg}}{\cancel{kg}} \quad x \quad \frac{1\ \cancel{kg}}{2.2\ \cancel{lb}} \quad x \quad \frac{242\ \cancel{lb}}{1}$$

$$= \quad \frac{\cancel{10}\ mL}{\underset{10}{\cancel{\underset{\cancel{500}}{\cancel{100}}}}} \quad x \quad \frac{\cancel{5}}{1} \quad x \quad \frac{1}{\underset{1}{\cancel{2.2}}} \quad x \quad \frac{\overset{110}{\cancel{242}}}{1}$$

$$= \quad \frac{110\ mL}{10}$$

$$= \quad 11\ mL$$

c. Ordered: 300 mL lactated Ringer's solution over 30 minutes
On hand: 1000 mL lactated Ringer's solution
Administration set: 10 gtt/mL

$$?gtt/min \quad = \quad \frac{10\ gtt}{1\ \cancel{mL}} \quad x \quad \frac{300\ \cancel{mL}}{30\ min}$$

$$= \quad \frac{\cancel{10}\ gtt}{1} \quad x \quad \frac{300}{\underset{3}{\cancel{30}}\ min}$$

$$= \quad \frac{\overset{100}{\cancel{300}}\ gtt}{3\ min}$$

$$= \quad 100\ gtt/min$$

d. Ordered: 1,000 mL normal saline over 4 hours
On hand: 1,000 mL normal saline
Administration set: 15 gtt/mL

$$?gtt/min \quad = \quad \frac{15\ gtt}{1\ \cancel{mL}} \quad x \quad \frac{1000\ \cancel{mL}}{4\ \cancel{hr}} \quad x \quad \frac{1\ \cancel{hr}}{60\ min}$$

$$= \quad \frac{\overset{1}{\cancel{15}}\ gtt}{1} \quad x \quad \frac{\overset{250}{\cancel{1000}}}{\underset{1}{\cancel{4}}} \quad x \quad \frac{1}{\underset{4}{\cancel{60}}\ min}$$

$$= \quad \frac{1\ gtt}{1} \quad x \quad \frac{250}{1} \quad x \quad \frac{1}{4\ min}$$

$$= \quad \frac{250\ gtt}{4\ min}$$

$$= \quad 62.5\ gtt/min \quad = \quad 63\ gtt/min$$

5. Patient is receiving 100 mg MSO$_4$ in 500 mL at 30 mL/hr.
How many mg/hr is the patient receiving?

$$?mg/hr \quad = \quad \frac{100\ mg}{500\ mL} \quad x \quad \frac{30\ mL}{1\ hr}$$

$$= \quad \frac{100\ mg}{500\ \cancel{mL}} \quad x \quad \frac{30\ \cancel{mL}}{1\ hr}$$

$$= \quad \frac{30\ mg}{5\ hr}$$

$$= \quad \frac{6\ mg}{1\ hr}$$

$$= \quad 6\ mg/hr$$

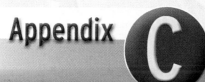

Appendix C

Sample Protocol

A protocol is an example of offline medical control—a procedure established to speed patient care when contact with direct medical control is impossible or impractical. Protocols are issued by individual counties and therefore differ depending on your work location. Because the protocol for your area may vary from this sample, the sample protocol should serve as reference only and should not be used when you are performing medical work.

Sample Procedure Protocol

VASCULAR ACCESS DEVICES

Special Information Needed

A. Obtain pertinent medical history if possible.

B. Obtain any information possible regarding the type of Vascular Access Device (VAD), number of lumens, purpose of the VAD, etc.

Indications

A. To obtain rapid venous access for the critical patient when peripheral access cannot be obtained.

Precautions

A. Obtain information and assistance from family members or home health professionals who are familiar with the device.

B. Discontinue any intermittent or continuous infusion pumps.

C. Assure placement and patency of the VAD prior to infusing any fluids or medications.

D. Flush the catheter completely with sterile normal saline.

E. Use aseptic technique.

Central Venous Catheters or PICC Lines

A. Attempt peripheral external jugular or intraosseous access first unless patient or patient's family insist on the direct usage of VAD.

B. Identify the location and type of VAD (i.e., central venous catheter, peripheral inserted central catheter).

C. Utilize knowledgeable family members, significant others, or home visiting nurse if available.

D. Discontinue and/or disconnect any pumps or medications.

E. Clamp the VAD closed to prevent air embolus.

F. If multiple lumen, identify the lumen to be used.

G. Utilize aseptic technique.

H. Briskly wipe the injection cap with an alcohol and/or povidone-iodine pad.

I. Insert the needle (attached to syringe) into the cap. Aspirate slowly for a positive blood return. Obtain blood samples if necessary. Then flush the line with solution.

J. Insert the needle (attached to a medication syringe or IV tubing) and infuse medications or fluids.

K. Secure the IV tubing.

L. Reassess the infusion site.

M. Reassess patient condition.

Implanted Ports

A. Attempt peripheral, external jugular, or intraosseous access first unless patient or patient's family insist on the direct usage of the VAD.

B. Identify the location and type of VAD (e.g., implanted port).

C. Utilize knowledgeable family members, significant others, or home visiting nurse if available.

D. Discontinue and/or disconnect any pumps or medications.

E. Carefully palpate the location of the implanted port.

F. If multiple ports, identify the port to be used.

G. Using sterile technique, prep the site with alcohol and/or povidone iodine. Wipe from the center outward three times in a circular motion.

H. Using a sterile gloved hand, press the skin firmly around the edges of the port.

I. Using a syringe filled with solution, insert the needle perpendicular to the skin.

J. Aspirate slowly for blood return, then flush the port prior to infusion.

K. Secure the IV tubing.

L. Reassess the infusion site.

M. Reassess the patient.

Complications

A. Patients with VADs are very susceptible to site infection or sepsis. Use sterile techniques at all times.

B. Sluggish flow or no flow may indicate a thrombosis. If a thrombosis is suspected, do not utilize the lumen.

C. Rarely, a catheter will migrate. The symptoms may include the following:
   1. burning with infusion
   2. site bleeding
   3. shortness of breath
   4. chest pain
   5. tachycardia and/or
   6. hypotension

If a catheter migration is suspected, do not use the VAD and treat the patient according to symptoms.

D. Catheters are durable but may leak or be torn. Extravasation of fluids or medications occurs and may cause burning and tissue damage. Clamp the catheter and do not use.

E. Air embolism may occur if the VAD is not clamped between infusions. Avoid this by properly clamping the catheter and preventing air from entering the system.

Sample Procedure Protocol

VENOUS ACCESS TECHNIQUE

GENERAL PRINCIPLES

Indications
A. Administer fluids for volume expansion

B. Administer drugs

Precautions
A. Do not start IVs distal to a fracture site or through skin damaged with more than erythema or superficial abrasion.

B. Due to the uncontrolled environment in which prehospital IVs are started, take extra care to use sterile technique.

C. Due to the high complication rate associated with prehospital IV therapy, use good judgment when deciding which patients should receive an IV.

Technique
A. Connect tubing to IV solution bag.

B. Fill drip chamber one-half full by squeezing.

C. Tear sufficient tape to anchor IV in place.

D. Use BSI precautions.

E. For pediatric patients, consider applying an arm board or splint prior to venipuncture.

F. **Scrub** insertion site with alcohol or iodine pads.

G. Don't palpate, unless necessary, after prep.

H. Perform venipuncture or enter bone marrow as described in the specific techniques described in this protocol.

I. After the catheter is in place, remove the needle or stylet and connect tubing.

J. Open full to check flow and placement, then slow to TKO rate unless otherwise indicated or ordered.

K. Secure tubing with tape, making sure of at least one 180-degree turn in the tubing when taping to be sure any traction on the tubing is not transmitted to the cannula itself.

L. Anchor with arm board or splint as needed to minimize chance of losing line with movement.

M. Recheck to be sure IV rate is as desired.

Complications

A. Pyrogenic reactions due to contaminated fluids become evident in about 30 minutes after starting the IV. Patient will develop fever, chills, nausea, vomiting, headache, backache, or general malaise. If observed, stop and remove IV immediately. Save the solution so it may be cultured.

B. Local: hematoma formation, infection, thrombosis, phlebitis. Note: the incidence of phlebitis is particularly high in the leg. Avoid use of lower extremity if possible.

C. Systemic: sepsis, pulmonary embolus, catheter fragment embolus, fiber embolus from solution in IV.

Side effects and special notes

A. Antecubital veins are useful access sites for patients in shock, but if possible, avoid areas near joints (or splint well!).

B. The point between the junction of two veins is more stable and often easier to use.

C. Start distally, and if successive attempts are necessary, you will be able to make more proximal attempts on the same vein without extravasating IV fluid.

D. Venipuncture itself is seldom morbid; however, the excess fluids that inadvertently run in when nobody is watching can be fatal!

E. The most difficult problem with IV insertion is knowing when to try and when to stop trying. Valuable time is often wasted attempting IVs when a critical patient requires blood. IV solutions may "buy time," but they frequently lose time instead. Generally, one attempt at the scene may be worthwhile, with a second attempt en route during long transports, if the patient is critical.

F. For the purpose of this protocol, peripheral IV will be defined as extremity or external jugular vein.

BUFF CAP (SALINE LOCK)

Indications

A. Prophylactic IV access

B. Drug administration

Precautions

A. Consider the patient, and whether a running IV or a buff cap is needed.

B. For any buff cap established in the prehospital setting, the attendant is responsible for showing the buff cap to the receiving nurse.

Technique

A. Assemble the necessary equipment.

B. Prefill the saline lock with sodium chloride.

C. Proceed with the technique for extremity IVs.

D. Remove the needle from the catheter and insert the saline lock.

E. Flush the saline lock with 2 to 5 mL of sodium chloride.

Contraindications

A. Any catheter placed in the external jugular vein

B. Any patient who is in need of fluid or is hypotensive

C. The cardiac arrest patient

EXTERNAL JUGULAR VEIN

Indications

A. Inability to secure extremity IV access

Technique

A. Position the patient: supine, head down (this may not be necessary or desirable if congestive heart failure or respiratory distress present). Turn patient's head opposite side of procedure.

B. Align the cannula in the direction of the vein, with the point aimed toward the ipsilateral shoulder (on the same side).

C. "Tourniquet" the vein lightly with one finger above the clavicle and apply traction to the skin above the angle of the jaw.

D. Make puncture midway between the angle of the jaw and the midclavicular line, "tourniqueting" the vein lightly with one finger above the clavicle.

E. Puncture the skin with the bevel of the needle upward; enter the vein either from the side or from above.

F. Note blood return and advance the catheter over the needle and remove "tourniquet."

EXTREMITY

Technique

A. Apply tourniquet proximal to proposed site to venous return only.

B. Hold vein in place by applying gentle traction on vein distal to point of entry.

C. Puncture the skin (with the bevel of the needle upward) about 0.5 to 1 cm from the vein and enter the vein either from the side or from above.

D. Note blood return and advance the catheter over the needle and remove tourniquet.

INTRAOSSEOUS INFUSION

Indications (Must meet all criteria)

A. Children less than 5 years old

B. Shock, cardiac arrest, status seizure

C. Unable to start peripheral line after one attempt; peripheral IV is always attempted first, intraosseous second. If in visual inspection unable to see good peripheral, go straight to intraosseous infusion.

D. Paramedics and Intermediates may insert intraosseous catheters.

Technique

A. Site of choice—tibia—one finger breadth below the tuberosity on the anteromedial surface

B. Clean skin with povidone iodine.

C. Place intraosseous needle perpendicular to the bone.

D. Apply firm downward pressure on the needle. A "screwing motion" facilitates advancement of the needle. Entrance into the bone marrow is indicated by a sudden loss of resistance.

E. Even if properly placed, the needle will not be secure. The needle must be secured and the IV tubing taped. The IO needle should be stabilized at all times. A person should be assigned to monitor the IV at the scene and en route to the hospital.

F. Only one intraosseous attempt is to be done in each tibia.

G. Puncture site to be covered with a dressing

Complications

A. Bone fracture (pushing too hard while not twisting the needle enough)

B. Infection

Contraindications

A. Fractures

B. Cellulitis

C. Osteogenesis imperfecta

Side effects and special notes

A. Some authorities recommend aspiration of marrow fluid or tissue to confirm needle location. This is not recommended for field procedures, as it increases the risk of plugging the needle.

B. The drugs and fluids that can be infused include: NaCl, epinephrine, atropine, lidocaine, dopamine, and Valium.

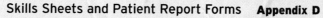

Appendix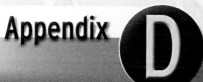

Skills Sheets and Patient Report Forms

These forms are examples of how to present and monitor IV therapy skills in the lab.

Student _____   Student ID Number _____

Evaluator _____   Date _____

Peripheral IV Technique and Insertion Skill Sheet	POINTS POSSIBLE	POINTS AWARDED
1. Takes or verbalizes BSI precautions	1	

2. Checks selected IV fluid for:
   Proper fluid (*1 point*)
   Fluid clarity (*1 point*)
	2	

3. Selects appropriate catheter	1	
4. Selects proper administration set	1	
5. Connects IV tubing to the IV bag	1	
6. Prepares administration set (fills drip chamber and flushes tubing)	1	
7. Cuts or tears tape (at any time before venipuncture)	1	
8. Applies constricting band	1	
9. Palpates suitable vein	1	
10. Cleanses site appropriately	1	

11. Performs venipuncture:
   Inserts catheter and needle (*1 point*)
   Notes or verbalizes flashback (*1 point*)
   Occludes vein proximal to catheter (*1 point*)
   Removes catheter needle (*1 point*)
   Connects IV tubing (*1 point*)
	5	

12. Releases constricting band	1	
13. Runs IV for brief period to assure patent line	1	
14. Secures catheter (tapes securely or verbalizes)	1	
15. Adjusts flow rate as appropriate	1	
16. Disposes/verbalizes disposal of needle in proper container	1	
Total	**21**	

Critical Criteria

_____ Did not take, or verbalize, body substance precautions.

_____ Exceeded the 6-minute time limit in establishing a patent and properly adjusted IV

_____ Contaminated equipment or site without appropriately correcting situation

_____ Any improper techniques resulting in the potential for catheter shear or air embolism

_____ Failed to successfully establish IV within 3 attempts

_____ Failed to remove constricting band after completing IV insertion

_____ Failed to dispose/verbalize disposal of needle in proper container

Preceptor Section:

If there are specific concerns or issues regarding the student's performance, technique, or attitude, please take time to address those issues here so they can be acknowledged and corrected by the course coordinator and the student.

Issue or concern:

Preceptor signature: _____ Date: _____

Student response:

Student signature: _____ Date: _____

Resolution:

Coordinator signature: _____ Date: _____

Student _____ Student ID Number_____

Evaluator _____ Date _____

Blood Draw via Vacutainer	**Points Possible**	**Points Awarded**
1. Takes or verbalizes BSI precautions	1	
2. Explains procedure to patient	1	
3. Identifies the need for drawing a blood sample: Routine as part of IV initiation for blood testing in hospital (*1 point*) Blood glucose determination (*1 point*)	2	

With IV	**W/O IV**		
4. Initiates IV in normal manner	4. Checks equipment	1	
5. Removes catheter needle and attaches Vacutainer barrel to the Luer adapter on the catheter	5. Applies constricting band and palpates suitable vein; performs venipuncture with needle-equipped Vacutainer barrel	1	
6. Fills Vacutainer tubes completely as vacuum dictates		1	
7. Gently inverts tubes with additives repeatedly (at least 10 times)		1	
8. Places tubes into small biohazard bag, labels the bag with patient's name, and secures bag with patient		1	
9. Secures IV or dresses puncture site		1	
10. Documents the procedure		1	
11. Disposes/verbalizes disposal of needle in proper container		1	
Total		12	

Critical Criteria

_____ Did not take, or verbalize, body substance precautions

_____ Exceeded the 6-minute time limit in establishing a patent IV and then drawing blood

_____ Contaminated equipment or site without appropriately correcting situation

_____ Any improper techniques resulting in the potential for catheter shear or air embolism

_____ Failed to label blood tubes

_____ Failed to dispose/verbalize disposal of needle in proper container

Preceptor Section:

If there are specific concerns or issues regarding the student's performance, technique, or attitude, please take time to address those issues here so they can be acknowledged and corrected by the course coordinator and the student.

Issue or concern:

Preceptor signature: _____ Date: _____

Student response:

Student signature: _____ Date: _____

Resolution:

Coordinator signature: _____ Date: _____

Student _____ Student ID Number _____

Evaluator _____ Date _____

D₅₀ (Dextrose 50%) Administration	POINTS POSSIBLE	POINTS AWARDED
1. Takes or verbalizes body substance isolation precautions	1	
2. Completes assessment(s) and determines that patient needs medication	1	
3. Calls medical direction for order or confirms standing order	1	
4. Lists indications for D₅₀ use: Hypoglycemia (*1 point*) Unconscious patient secondary to unknown etiology (*1 point*) Non-traumatic seizures (*1 point*) Glucometer reading <70 mg/dL (*1 point*)	4	
5. Checks for known allergies, contraindications or incompatibilities: Seizures secondary to trauma (*1 point*) Extravasation and tissue necrosis (*1 point*) Questionable use in CVA patients (*1 point*) Requires a pre-administration blood sample to be drawn (*1 point*)	4	
6. Checks medication to determine: Expiration date (*1 point*) Concentration (*1 point*) Correctness (*1 point*) Clarity (*1 point*)	4	
7. Lists the appropriate dosage for the medication: Adult: 25 g slow IV (*1 point*) Peds: 2 to 4 mL /kg of D₂₅ (1 to 6 years of age) (*1 point*) 2 to 4 mL/kg of D₁₀ (<1 year of age) (*1 point*)	3	
8. Properly administers medication: Draws up required dosage (*1 point*) Instructs patient about the medications effects (*1 point*) Administers medication in IV port—slow push (*1 point*) Periodically flows IV to ensure patency of line (*1 point*) Follows medication with a saline bolus/flush (20 mL) (*1 point*)	5	
9. Verbalizes the need for transport	1	
10. Verbalizes ongoing assessment including observing patient for desired/adverse side effects	1	
11. Voices proper documentation of medication administration	1	
Total	26	

Critical Criteria

_____ Did not take, or verbalize, body substance precautions.

_____ Did not complete, or verbalize completion of, patient assessment.

_____ Administered medication without physician order.

_____ Administered, or attempted to administer, a medication to a patient with one or more contraindications for use.

_____ Administered improper medication dosage (wrong drug, incorrect amount, or pushed at an inappropriate rate).

Preceptor Section:

If there are specific concerns or issues regarding the student's performance, technique, or attitude, please take time to address those issues here so they can be acknowledged and corrected by the course coordinator and the student.

Issue or concern:

Preceptor signature: _____ Date: _____

Student response:

Student signature: _____ Date: _____

Resolution:

Coordinator signature: _____ Date: _____

Student _____ Student ID Number _____

Evaluator _____ Date _____

Glucometer Skill Sheet	Points Possible	Points Awarded
1. Takes or verbalizes BSI precautions	1	
2. Identifies the need for obtaining a blood glucose level: Altered level of consciousness (*1 point*) Suspected diabetic (*1 point*) Non-traumatic seizures (*1 point*) Unconscious patient of unknown etiology (*1 point*)	4	
3. Identifies the normal parameters for blood glucose (70 to 120 mg/dL)	1	
4. Identifies contraindications: None (*1 point*)	1	
5. Identifies potential complications: Erroneous readings (excessively low <20 mg/dL or high >200 mg/dL) (*1 point*) Potential exposure to pathogens (*1 point*) Arterial sample (*1 point*) Clotted blood sample (*1 point*)	4	
6. Checks equipment: Glucometer machine (*1 point*) Test strip (*1 point*) Needle or spring-loaded puncture device (*1 point*) Alcohol prep(s) (*1 point*)	4	
7. Explains procedure to patient	1	
8. Turns on power to machine	1	
9. Preps finger tip with alcohol	1	
10. Lances the prepped site with needle/lancet device, drawing blood	1	
11. Expresses blood sample and transfers it to test strip	1	
12. Dresses puncture site	1	
13. Records reading from monitor and documents it appropriately	1	
14. Disposes/verbalizes disposal of needle/lancet in appropriate container	1	
Total	23	

Critical Criteria

_____ Did not take, or verbalize, body substance precautions

_____ Failed to identify 2 indications

_____ Failed to identify 2 potential complications

_____ Failed to identify normal parameters

_____ Failed to dispose of needle/lancet in an appropriate container

Preceptor Section:

If there are specific concerns or issues regarding the student's performance, technique, or attitude, please take time to address those issues here so they can be acknowledged and corrected by the course coordinator and the student.

Issue or concern:

Preceptor signature: _____ Date: _____

Student response:

Student signature: _____ Date: _____

Resolution:

Coordinator signature: _____ Date: _____

Student _____   Student ID Number _____

Evaluator _____   Date _____

Butterfly Vein Cannulation	Points Possible	Points Awarded
1. Takes or verbalizes BSI precautions	1	
2. Checks selected IV fluid for: Proper fluid (*1 point*) Clarity (*1 point*) Expiration (*1 point*)	3	
3. Selects appropriate equipment to include: Butterfly needle (*1 point*) Syringe (*1 point*) Saline (*1 point*) Extension tubing (*1 point*) Constricting band (*1 point*)	5	
4. Selects proper administration set (volutrol burette)	1	
5. Connects administration set/volutrol to bag	1	
6. Prepares administration set (fills drip chamber and flushes tubing)	1	
7. Prepares syringe and extension tubing	1	
8. Cuts or tears tape (at any time before venipuncture)	1	
9. Identifies proper anatomical site for venipuncture	1	
10. Cleanses site appropriately	1	
11. Performs venipuncture: Applies constricting band (*1 point*) Inserts needle at proper angle (*1 point*) Advances needle until "pop" is felt (*1 point*) Takes care to avoid any infiltration or needle movement (*1 point*)	4	
12. Attaches syringe and extension set to butterfly needle	1	
13. Aspirates blood sample to confirm placement/obtain blood sample	1	
14. Releases venous constricting band	1	
15. Slowly injects saline to assure proper placement of needle	1	
16. Connects administration set and adjusts flow rate as appropriate	1	
17. Secures needle with tape	1	
Total	26	

Critical Criteria

_____ Failed to take or verbalize BSI precautions prior to performing venipuncture

_____ Failed to establish a patent and properly adjusted line within the time limit

_____ Contaminated equipment or site without appropriately correcting situation

_____ Any improper technique resulting in the potential for air embolism

_____ Failed to assure correct needle placement before attaching administration set

_____ Failed to establish vein infusion successfully within 2 attempts

_____ Performed scalp venipuncture in an unacceptable manner
(improper puncture site, incorrect needle angle, etc.)

Preceptor Section:

If there are specific concerns or issues regarding the student's performance, technique, or attitude, please take time to address those issues here so they can be acknowledged and corrected by the course coordinator and the student.

Issue or concern:

Preceptor signature: _____ Date: _____

Student response:

Student signature: _____ Date: _____

Resolution:

Coordinator signature: _____ Date: _____

IV Therapy Training Report Form *(Not intended as actual patient reporting tool)*

EMS Call Information:

Location of Call

Destination Facility

Call Personnel	Type of Call:	Response to Call:	Times:
Driver:	____ Medical	____ Emergent	Enroute:
Attendant:	____ Trauma	____ Non-emergent	Arrival:
3rd Rider:	____ Assist	**Response to Facility:**	Out:
Other Agency Response:	____ Other	____ Emergent	Cleared:
		____ Non-emergent	Cancelled:

Patient Information:

Name:

Chief Complaint:

Medications:

Medical Hx: Allergies:

Patient Vitals:

Time	Pulse	Blood Pressure	Resp. Rate	Breath Sounds	Pupils	Skin	Glasgow Coma Scale O V M	Circulation, sensation, movement of extremities (explain any NO in report)			
								L Arm R		L Leg R	
:		/						Yes No	Yes No	Yes No	Yes No
:		/						Yes No	Yes No	Yes No	Yes No
:		/						Yes No	Yes No	Yes No	Yes No
:		/						Yes No	Yes No	Yes No	Yes No

Patient Procedures/Medications:

Time	Procedure	Time	Medication	Dose	Route	ECG Rhythm
:		:				
:		:				
:		:				
:		:				

Patient Report:

_____

_____

_____

_____

_____

EMT Name: _____ Date: _____

Preceptor Name: _____ Date: _____

Preceptor Section:

If there are specific concerns or issues regarding the student's performance, technique, or attitude, please take time to address those issues here so they can be acknowledged and corrected by the course coordinator and the student.

Issue or concern:

Preceptor signature: _____ Date: _____

Student response:

Student signature: _____ Date: _____

Resolution:

Coordinator signature: _____ Date: _____

Appendix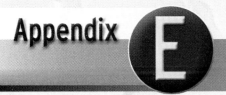

IV Skills Check-Off Sheet

The following form is an example that can be used in the laboratory portion of the course for evaluation on a practice or live arm. Students should read the evaluation sheet and understand the rationale for each criterion. If any requirements are unclear, it is the responsibility of the student to obtain clarification before attempting any practice sticks. Students should not pass the laboratory portion of the course until they can meet the critical criteria listed on the form and demonstrate adequate intravenous skills.

IV Skills Check-Off Sheet

Student Name _____

Skills Preceptor Name:	PASS	RETEST
1. Takes BSI precautions		
2. Identifies need for IV		
3. Informs patient of procedure		
4. Gathers all equipment		
a. Checks bag for clarity, correct solution, and expiration		
b. Chooses correct IV drip set		
c. Spikes bag using aseptic technique		
d. Primes IV line and purges air out of tubing		
e. Assembles Luer adapters or has syringe closed for drawing blood		
f. Gathers all appropriate blood tubes for blood collection		
g. Tears IV tape in preparation for securing the IV site		
h. Has 4-inch x 4-inch gauze pads close by to absorb any blood spillage		
5. Identifies appropriate vein for catheter insertion		
6. Chooses correct size IV catheter for insertion		
7. Applies constricting band to patient's arm above the chosen IV site		
8. Cleans chosen site using either alcohol or iodine swabs		

Skills Preceptor Name:	Pass	Retest
9. Inserts catheter beveled side up		
10. Removes needle, leaving catheter in place		
11. Secures Vacutainer blood collection device or syringe into the end of the catheter		
12. Fills blood tubes in correct order or fills syringe without hemolysis		
13. Removes blood collection devices and tamponades vein		
14. Removes constricting band from patient's arm		
15. Attaches IV tubing to catheter end		
16. Opens IV stop cock to check for flow		
17. Evaluates IV site for IV patency		
18. Adjusts IV flow rate to desired delivery rate		
19. Secures IV tubing and catheter with IV tape		
20. Administers medication according to protocol		
21. Checks and monitors patient and vital signs for changes		
22. Discontinues IV line according to protocol		
23. Documents entire procedure on trip report		

Critical Criteria: *Any missed item constitutes practical failure*	Failed
Student failed to use BSI	
Student failed to use aseptic technique	
Student left constricting band in place too long before beginning IV insertion	
Student did not visualize and adjust IV flow rate after procedure	
Student left constricting band around arm after procedure completed	

Preceptor Section:

If there are specific concerns or issues regarding the student's performance, technique, or attitude, please take time to address those issues here so that they can be acknowledged and corrected by the course coordinator and the student.

Issue or concern:

Preceptor signature: _____   Date: _____

Student response:

Student signature: _____   Date: _____

Resolution:

Coordinator signature: _____   Date: _____

Appendix

IV Starts Log Sheet

The following log sheet is an example provided to record your practice arm sticks, IV starts on lab partners, and field IV starts.

IV Starts Log

Student Name:_____

IV Instructor:_____

Start Date:_____

****Print all information****

	Patient ID #	Preceptor (Name/Title/Agency)	Preceptor Signature
1. Lab stick			
2. Lab stick			
3. Lab stick			
4. Lab stick			
5. Live stick			
6. Live stick			
7.			
8.			
9.			
10.			

Glossary

abandonment: The termination of patient care without assuring the continuation of that care at the same medical level or higher.

absolute contraindication: A situation in which a treatment should never be used.

access port: A sealed hub on an administration set designed for sterile access to the IV fluid.

acid: Any molecule that gives up a hydrogen ion; often referred to as H^+.

acidosis: A pathologic condition resulting from the accumulation of acids in the body.

acquired immune deficiency syndrome (AIDS): An illness caused by the human immunodeficiency virus (HIV). AIDS affects the immune system of the body by destroying the cells that control and initiate an immune response.

activated charcoal: Charcoal ground into a very fine powder that provides the greatest possible surface area for binding drugs that have been taken by mouth; it is carried on the EMS unit.

acts allowed: The tasks that an EMT is allowed to perform, as defined by the state EMS regulatory agency and physician advisory.

actual fluid loss: The actual loss of fluid from the vascular compartment of the body.

actual hypovolemia: The term used to describe fluid movement out of the vascular compartment.

acute myocardial infarction: Heart attack; death of the heart muscle following obstruction of blood flow to it. Acute in this context means "new" or "happening right now."

administration set: Tubing that connects to the IV bag access port and the catheter in order to deliver the IV fluid.

advance directive: Written documentation that specifies medical treatment for a competent patient should the patient become unable to make decisions.

advanced life support (ALS): Advanced lifesaving procedures, such as cardiac monitoring, starting IV fluids, giving medications, and using advanced airway adjuncts.

aerobic cellular respiration: Cellular metabolism of glucose in the presence of oxygen.

agonal respirations: An irregular, gasping respiration, sometimes heard in dying patients.

air embolus: The presence of air in the veins, which can lead to cardiac arrest if it enters the lungs.

alcohol withdrawal syndrome: A set of signs and symptoms brought on when a person who abuses alcohol on a chronic basis suddenly stops consuming alcohol. It includes tremors, hallucinations, and CNS problems.

alcoholic ketoacidosis: The metabolic acidotic state that manifests from the poor nutritional habits of chronic alcohol abuse. Both the liver and the body experience inadequate fuel reserves of glycogen and thus have to switch to fatty acid metabolism.

alkalosis: A pathologic condition resulting from the accumulation of bases in the body.

altered level of consciousness: Any state of consciousness that differs from what is considered a normal state of consciousness. An altered LOC can be present in any age group.

anaerobic cellular respiration: Cellular metabolism of glucose in the absence of oxygen. This is a defensive, emergency form of metabolism.

anaphylactic shock: Severe shock caused by an allergic reaction.

anaphylaxis: An extreme, life-threatening systemic allergic reaction that may include shock and respiratory failure.

aneurysm: A swelling or enlargement of a part of an artery, resulting from weakening of the arterial wall.

anion: An ion that contains an overall negative charge.

antecubital: The anterior aspect of the elbow.

anticoagulant: A substance that prevents blood from clotting.

antidiuretic hormone (ADH): A hormone produced by the pituitary gland that signals the kidneys to prevent excretion of water.

arteriovenous shunt (AV shunt): A surgical opening between an artery and a vein to allow dialysis access.

assault: The threat of injury directed at either the patient or the EMT.

asystole: Complete absence of cardiac electrical activity.

ataxia: A staggered walk or gait caused by injury to the brain or spinal cord.

auscultation: A method of listening to sounds within an organ with a stethoscope.

automated external defibrillator (AED): A machine that can administer an electrical shock to the heart if needed.

autonomic nervous system: The part of the nervous system that regulates involuntary functions, such as digestion and sweating. The two major divisions of the autonomic nervous system are the sympathetic and parasympathetic nervous systems.

AVPU scale: A method of assessing a patient's level of consciousness by determining whether a patient is awake and alert, responsive to verbal stimulus or pain, or unresponsive, used principally in the initial assessment.

barbiturate: A class of drugs that acts as a sedative that induces sleep.

base: Any molecule that can accept a hydrogen ion; often referred to as OH^-.

basic life support (BLS): Noninvasive emergency lifesaving care that is used to treat airway obstruction, respiratory arrest, or cardiac arrest.

battery: The physical contact that occurs illegally between an EMT and a patient unless permission for treatment has been given by the patient.

biohazard bag: A bag designed to hold discarded materials that have been contaminated with body fluids or other potentially dangerous substances.

blood pump: A macrodrip IV set that also has a mechanical pump to aid in the infusion of fluid into a patient.

blood tubing: A special type of macrodrip IV set intended for rapid blood and/or fluid resuscitation of a patient.

blow: A term that refers to the extravasation of an IV site.

blunt trauma: A mechanism of injury in which force occurs over a broad area, and the skin is not usually broken.

body substance isolation (BSI): An infection control concept and practice that assumes that all body fluids are potentially infectious.

bradypnea: Slow respiratory rate.

buffer: A substance or group of substances that controls the hydrogen levels in a solution.

bunker gear: Protective outerwear that acts as a heat and moisture barrier and is worn by fire response agencies and some EMS agencies.

butterfly catheter: A rigid, hollow, venous cannulation device identified by its plastic "wings" that act as anchoring points for securing the catheter.

cannulation: The insertion of a hollow tube into a vein to allow for fluid flow.

capillary beds: The terminal ends of the vascular system where fluids, food, and wastes are exchanged between the vascular system and the cells of the body.

capillary refill: A test that evaluates the ability of the circulatory system to restore blood to the capillary system.

cardiac arrest: A state in which the heart fails to generate an effective and detectible blood flow; pulses are not palpable in cardiac arrest, even if muscular and electrical activity continues in the heart.

cardiac dysrhythmia: An abnormal cardiac rhythm.

cardiogenic shock: A state in which not enough oxygen is delivered to the tissues of the body, caused by low output of blood from the heart. It can be a severe complication of a large acute myocardial infarction, as well as other conditions.

cardiotoxic: Any substance that is harmful or toxic to the heart.

carotid pulse: The pulse taken at the carotid artery—the major artery in the neck that supplies blood to the head and brain.

carpal/pedal spasms: Hand/foot spasms.

catheter: A flexible, hollow structure that drains or delivers fluids.

catheter shear: The cutting of the catheter by the laser sharpened needle during improper cannulation technique; the severed piece can then enter the circulatory system.

cation: An ion that contains an overall positive charge.

cellular metabolism: The process by which cells take in substrates like glucose and oxygen to create ATP for energy.

cellular perfusion: The ability of a cell to take in and maintain water levels.

central nervous system (CNS) depression: The slowing of the nervous system function of the brain secondary to delays in nerve cell transmission. Several factors can influence CNS depressions, including nerve cell permeability, hypoxia, drugs, and injury.

central pulse: Pulses that can be assessed in core areas like the femoral artery and carotid artery.

centrifuge: A machine that rotates at 10,000 to 15,000 rpm to separate fluid components into layers by weight.

cerebral edema: Swelling of the brain.

cerebral ischemia: Poor blood flow through cerebral arteries due to some form of blockage or occlusion.

cerebral perfusion: The ability of fluid to move from cerebral circulation to cerebral tissue, carrying oxygen and nutrients to the cells.

cerebral vasodilation: Enlargement of cerebral blood vessels.

cerebrovascular accident (CVA): The interruption of blood flow to the brain that results in the loss of brain function.

cirrhosis: Destruction of liver tissue secondary to infections or toxic exposures.

closed head injury: Injury usually associated with trauma in which the brain has been injured but the skin has not been broken, and there is no obvious bleeding.

clotting factors: An elaborate collection of substrates and proteins that combine to control and stop bleeding; often, one of the first steps in the clotting cascade.

compensated stage: The early stage of shock, while the body can still compensate for blood loss.

competent: Able to make rational decisions about personal well-being.

complex partial seizure: A type of simple seizure that does begin to affect a person's level of consciousness

concentration gradient: The natural tendency for substances to flow from an area of higher concentration to an area of lower concentration, either within the cell or outside the cell.

congestive heart failure: A disorder in which the heart loses its ability to pump blood effectively, usually as a result of damage to the heart muscle, and usually resulting in a back-up of fluid into the lungs.

contaminated stick: The puncturing of an emergency care provider's skin with a catheter that was used on a patient.

contraindication: Situation in which a drug should not be given because it would not help or may actually harm a patient.

crackles: The "crackling" sound heard by air moving through fluid-filled alveolar sacs.

cross-contamination: The ability to spread possible infection from one individual to another by the exchange of contaminated body fluids. The greatest risks for cross-contamination occur when proper BSI precautions are ignored or overlooked.

crystalloid solution: A type of intravenous solution that contains compounds that quickly disassociate in solution and can cross membranes. Crystalloid solutions are considered the best choice for prehospital care of injured patients who need fluids to replace lost body fluid.

D$_5$W: 5% dextrose in water.

date rape drugs: A class of drugs used to incapacitate an individual; these drugs are seen with increasing frequency in cases of "date rape" and sexual assaults.

"daydream" seizure: A petit mal seizure in which a patient becomes flaccid and stares into space.

depolarization: The rapid movement of electrolytes across a cell membrane that changes the cell's overall charge. This rapid shifting of electrolytes and cellular charges is the main catalyst for muscle contractions and neural transmissions.

diabetes insipidus: A form of diabetes characterized by polyuria and polydipsia (excessive thirst) that often results from decreased or absent ADH production.

diabetic ketoacidosis (DKA): A form of acidosis in uncontrolled diabetes; an excess accumulation of certain acids that occurs when insulin is not available in the body.

diaphoresis: Excessive sweating.

diffusion: A process in which molecules move from an area of higher concentration to an area of lower concentration.

dimensional analysis: A calculation method in which relationships are set up in equations so that like units can be canceled out.

diphtheria: An infectious disease in which a membrane lining the pharynx develops that can severely obstruct passage of air into the larynx.

disassociate: To lose a hydrogen atom in the presence of water. Acids are classified as either strong or weak, depending on how completely they disassociate in water.

distributive shock: A category of shock which results from poor distribution of fluids in the body. This category includes neurogenic, septic, anaphylactic, and obstructive shock.

diuresis: Fluid loss caused by diuretic medications or a medical condition such as diabetic ketoacidosis.

do not resuscitate order (DNR): Written documentation giving permission to medical personnel not to attempt resuscitation in the event of cardiac arrest.

drip chamber: The area of the administration set where fluid accumulates so that the tubing remains filled with fluid.

drip rate: Number of drops per minute.

drip set: Another name for an administration set.

durable medical power of attorney: Written documentation that directs someone to act on behalf of the patient regarding medical treatment.

dyspnea: Shortness of breath or difficulty breathing.

edema: The presence of abnormally large amounts of fluid in the extracellular spaces of body tissues, causing swelling of the affected area.

electrolyte: A charged atom or compound that results from the loss or gain of an electron. Electrolytes are ions that the body uses to perform certain critical metabolic processes.

epi dump: A term used to describe a rapid epinephrine infusion into the blood.

epicardium: The smooth outer layer of the heart.

epidural bleeding: A life-threatening hemorrhage that develops between the brain and the skull; shearing and tearing of the arteries above the dural lining of the brain allow blood to escape into the cavity and compress the brain.

epilepsy: An idiopathic neurological disease that produces rapid and sudden electrical discharges in the brain.

epinephrine: A substance (adrenaline) produced by the body and a drug produced by pharmaceutical companies to increase pulse and blood pressure; the drug of choice for an anaphylactic reaction.

erythrocytes: Red blood cells (RBCs).

esophageal varices: Chronic irritation of esophageal tissue resulting in exposed vasculature susceptible to rupture and possibly fatal blood loss.

evisceration: The displacement of organs outside the body.

external jugular IV: IV access established in the jugular veins of the neck.

extravasation: An escape of fluid such as blood, serum, or lymph fluid into the tissues.

extrication: Removal of a patient from entrapment or a dangerous situation or position, such as removal from a wrecked vehicle, industrial accident, or building collapse.

false imprisonment: The illegal detention of a patient against his or her will when transporting the person to the hospital.

fascia: The fiber-like connective tissue that covers arteries, veins, tendons, and ligaments.

fibrin: A water-insoluble gel that results from the combining of thrombin and fibrinogen and forms a scab.

fibrinogen: The substrate that is converted by thrombin into fibrin in the clotting process.

flash chamber: The area of a catheter that fills with blood to help indicate when a vein is cannulated.

fluid reserves: Areas in the body from which fluid can be "borrowed" to maintain vascular volume.

formed elements: The solid components of blood found in plasma. This category includes red blood cells, white blood cells, and platelets.

gauge: The interior diameter of the catheter.

generalized seizure: Seizure characterized by severe twitching of all the body's muscles that may last several minutes or more; also known as a grand mal seizure.

Glasgow coma scale: A method of evaluating a patient's neural functions by assessing three systems: eye opening, motor response, and verbal response.

glucagon: The hormone released from the alpha cells in the islets of Langerhans that converts glycogen back into glucose when the body's blood glucose levels drop.

glucometer: A device designed to measure circulating glucose levels.

gluconeogenesis: The process by which glycogen is converted back into glucose.

glycolysis: The conversion of glucose into energy via metabolic pathways.

gtt: A measurement that indicates drops per milliliter.

half-life: The time needed for a drug's circulating levels to reach one half its original dosage. Half-life times are critical in establishing and maintaining therapeutic drug levels for the patient.

HazMat containment: The act of minimizing possible exposure to a hazardous material. A hazardous material is defined as any substance that is toxic, poisonous, radioactive, flammable, or explosive, and causes injury or death with exposure.

heart rate: The wave of pressure that is created as the heart contracts and forces blood out of the left ventricle and into the major arteries.

heat cramps: Painful muscle spasms usually associated with vigorous activity in a hot environment.

heat exhaustion: A form of heat injury in which the body loses significant amounts of fluid and electrolytes from heavy sweating, which results in dizziness, nausea, confusion, collapse, and severe weakness; also called heat prostration or heat collapse.

hematocrit: A common lab test to measure the amounts of formed and unformed elements of the blood.

hematoma: An accumulation of blood in the tissues surrounding an IV site.

heme ring: A protein ring containing four ferrous (iron) atoms.

hemorrhagic shock: A specific form of hypovolemia that results from severe blood loss.

HEPAmask: A type of mask that prevents the wearer from inhaling airborne pathogens such as the tuberculosis bacterium.

hepatic encephalopathy: Destruction of cerebral cells and tissues as a result of increasing blood toxins secondary to hepatic failure.

hepatitis: An infection of the liver, usually caused by a virus, that causes fever, loss of appetite, jaundice, fatigue, and altered liver function.

homeostasis: The balance of all systems of the body; also known as homeostatic balance.

human immunodeficiency virus (HIV): A virus that can lead to infection and subsequently to acquired immune deficiency syndrome (AIDS).

huffer: A slang term for anyone who inhales fumes as a form of drug abuse.

hydrophilic: Water-loving.

hydrophobic: Water-fearing.

hyperresonance: The term used to describe the loud, clear breath sounds heard on auscultation when assessing a pneumothorax.

hypercalcemia: High calcium levels.

hyperglycemia: High circulating blood glucose levels.

hyperkalemia: High levels of potassium.

hypertension: Blood pressure that is higher than the normal range.

hypertonic: A solution that has a greater concentration of sodium than does the cell; the increased extracellular osmotic pressure can draw water out of the cell and cause it to collapse.

hyperventilation: A lowering of blood carbon dioxide levels, usually through rapid or deep breathing.

hypocalcemia: Low serum calcium levels.

hypoglycemia: Low circulating blood glucose levels.

hypokalemia: Low levels of potassium.

hypoperfusion: A condition that develops when the circulatory system is not able to deliver sufficient blood and oxygen to body organs, resulting in organ failure and eventual death if untreated.

hypotension: Blood pressure that is lower than the normal range.

hypothermia: A condition in which the internal body temperature falls below 95°F (35°C) after exposure to a cold environment.

hypotonic: A solution that has a lower concentration of sodium than does the cell; the increased intracellular osmotic pressure lets water flow into the cell, causing it to swell and possibly burst.

hypoventilation: Inadequate air movement in and out of the lungs resulting in decreased respiration.

hypovolemia: A state of shock that results when there is actual fluid loss from the body.

hypovolemic shock: Condition in which low blood volume from massive internal or external bleeding or extensive loss of body water results in inadequate perfusion.

hypoxemia: Low oxygen concentrations in blood cells.

hypoxia: A decreased amount of circulating oxygen in the blood, which can lead to cellular dysfunction and cellular death.

hypoxic drive: A "backup system" to control respiration.

idiopathic: Any disease process that has no identifiable causes or origins.

immunocompromised: The inability of the immune system to respond to an infection resulting from immunosuppressive medications given to transplant patients or disease processes like AIDS.

infarct: Death of a body tissue, usually caused by interruption of its blood supply.

infection: The abnormal invasion of a host or host tissue by organisms such as bacteria, viruses, or parasites, with or without signs or symptoms of disease.

infiltration: The escape of fluid into the surrounding tissue.

inoculant: An injected compound (usually a drug or medication) designed to illicit a favorable response from the immune system to control or prevent an illness.

insulin shock: Unconsciousness or altered mental status in a patient with diabetes caused by significant hypoglycemia; usually the result of excessive exercise and activity or failure to eat after a routine dose of insulin.

interstitial: Water between the vascular system and the surrounding cells (for example, between the membranes of two cells located outside the vascular compartment in the body).

intracranial bleeding: Accumulation of blood within cerebral tissue following some type of cerebral vascular injury.

intracranial pressure (ICP): Increased pressure within the cranial vault resulting from fluid accumulation outside the cerebral vascular compartment.

intraosseous: Into the bone; a medication delivery route.

intraosseous IV (IO): An IV that is placed into a bone.

intravascular: The water portion of the circulatory system surrounding the blood cells (for example in the heart, arteries, or veins).

ion: A charged atom or compound that results from the loss or gain of an electron.

ionic concentration: The amount of charged particles found in a particular area.

iron deficiency anemia: Reduction in the amount of available blood cells secondary to the decreased availability of iron needed to create hemoglobin.

irreversible stage: The final stage of shock, resulting in death.

ischemia: A lack of oxygen that deprives tissues of necessary nutrients, resulting from partial or complete blockage of blood flow.

islets of Langerhans: The beta cells found in the pancreas that are responsible for the production of insulin.

isotonic: A solution that has the same concentration of sodium as does the cell. In this case, water doesn't shift, and no change in cell shape occurs.

isotonic crystalloids: The main type of fluid used in the prehospital setting for fluid replacement because of its ability to support blood pressure by remaining within the vascular compartment.

IV push: A term used to describe a mode of medication administration through an established IV line.

Jacksonian seizure: A focal motor seizure presenting with muscle spasms in the patient, affecting only one side of the body.

Jamshedi needle: A type of intraosseous double needle consisting of a solid boring needle inside a sharpened hollow needle.

jugular vein distention (JVD): The visible bulging of the jugular veins when the patient is in semi-fowlers or full fowlers position. JVD is indicative of inadequate blood movement through the heart and/or lungs.

keep-the-vein-open IV set up: A phrase that refers to the flow rate of a maintenance IV line established as a prophylactic access.

ketoacidosis: An acidotic state created by the production of ketones via fat metabolism.

ketones: The byproducts of fat metabolism secondary to use of fatty acids rather than glucose by body cells. An excess of ketones can lead to ketoacidosis.

Kussmaul respirations: A breathing pattern characterized by rapid and deep respirations that develops after a patient's pH levels become acidotic.

lactated Ringer's solution (LR): A crystalloid isotonic intravenous solution that is generally not used in the field.

lactic acidosis: The metabolic acidotic state resulting from the accumulation of lactic acid secondary to anaerobic cellular metabolism.

level of consciousness (LOC): A measurement of just how aware a person is to the surroundings and situation.

living will: A legal document that expresses a patient's wishes regarding medical treatment should he or she become incompetent. This is much like an advance directive but this term is usually used when the document is completed by a competent patient who has not developed any medical disorders.

local reaction: Mild to moderate allergic reaction.

lysis: The rupturing of a cell caused by either the presence of certain enzymes or the uncontrolled influx of material into the cell.

lysosome: An intracellular structure that contains hydrogen peroxide and thus the ability to destroy cells upon release.

macrodrip set: An administration set named for the large orifice between the piercing spike and the drip chamber. A macrodrip set allows for rapid fluid flow into the vascular system.

macrophage: A large, primary response immune cell that polices the body and removes any damaged or foreign substances.

malfeasance: Wrongdoing that is illegal or contrary to official obligations.

manual infusion: The act of physically forcing fluid into the vascular compartment.

manual traction: One way an EMT can stabilize an IV access point by pulling the skin taut across the site.

meningitis: Inflammation of the meninges that covers the spinal cord and the brain.

mentation: A patient's thought process.

metabolic: The breakdown of ingested foodstuffs into smaller and smaller molecules and atoms that are used as energy sources for cellular function.

metabolic acidosis: A metabolic state of acidosis resulting from retention of H+ or other positively charged ions not related to respiratory compromise.

microdrip set: An administration set named for the small orifice between the piercing spike and the drip chamber. A microdrip set allows for carefully controlled fluid flow and is ideally suited for medication administration.

misfeasance: The improper and unlawful execution of some act that itself is lawful and proper.

mottling: Systemic pooling of blood due to circulatory failure.

mucosa: Mucous membrane layer.

mucous membranes: The lining of body cavities and passages that are in direct contact with the outside environment.

myocardial contusion: A bruise of the heart muscle.

narcotic: A class of drug derived from opium that acts as a hypnotic or painkiller such as codeine and morphine.

narrowing pulse pressure: The reduction of the gap between systolic and diastolic blood pressures, so that the systolic and diastolic pressures approach each other.

necrosis: Cellular destruction resulting in tissue death.

negligence: Deviation from the accepted standard of care that results in further injury to the patient.

neonate: Children who range in age from birth to one month.

neural permeability: The rate at which a nerve cell permits calcium to cross its cell membrane. Accelerated rates of calcium absorption lead to rapid, continual nerve impulse transmission while decelerated rates of calcium absorption lead to decreased nerve impulse transmission.

neural transmission: The speed at which an impulse travels through the nerve cell. The rate of transmission is directly related to neural permeability.

neurogenic shock: Circulatory failure caused by paralysis of the nerves that control the size of the blood vessels. Seen in spinal cord injuries.

nonfeasance: Failure to perform some act that is either an official duty or legal requirement.

nonformed element: The sticky, liquid portion of the blood; plasma.

obstructive shock: Produced when there is a physical blockage of the patient's circulation as seen with massive pulmonary embolus.

occlusion: Blockage, usually of a tubular structure such as a blood vessel.

opsite: A type of sterile covering for IV sites.

"orange peel" nose: An orange peel appearance to the skin of the nose, most commonly associated with chronic alcoholism.

organophosphates: A name given to specific chemical compounds found in pesticides and some forms of nerve gas. Organophosphates act as neurotoxins, blocking or inhibiting neural activity.

osmolarity: The ability to influence the movement of water across a semi-permeable membrane.

osmosis: The diffusion of water across a cell membrane.

osmotic pressure: Pressure created against the cell wall by the presence of water.

over-the-needle catheter: The prehospital standard for IV cannulation. It consists of a hollow tube over a laser-sharpened steel needle.

oxyhemoglobin: A structure formed when oxygen binds with the ferrous ring of hemoglobin.

pancreatitis: Inflammation of the pancreas.

parasympathetic stimulation: Part of the autonomic nervous system responsible for the vegetative/regenerative state of the body.

patient refusal: A verbalized wish from a patient indicating that he or she does not wish to be medically treated. Patient refusals must be documented by emergency medical personnel.

penrose drain: A type of surgical drain often used as a constricting band.

perceived fluid loss: Vasodilation of the vascular compartment that produces signs and symptoms mimicking actual fluid losses even though no fluid has been lost.

perceived hypovolemia: Dilation of the vasculature, resulting in a decreased circulating pressure and shock. This type of shock is not caused by actual fluid loss from the body.

perforation: The physical act of entering a vein. If not carefully monitored, the perforation can lead to extravasation.

perfusion: The circulation of blood within an organ or tissue in adequate amounts to meet the cells' current needs.

pericardial tamponade: Acute compression of the heart resulting from a buildup of blood or other fluid in the pericardium. The fluid accumulation begins to impede normal cardiac function and filling.

pericardium: The fibrous sac that surrounds the heart.

peripheral circulation: Circulation that is outside the core areas of the body, such as in the extremities.

peripheral IV: Any intravenous access established in the venous circulation that is not part of the patient's central circulation.

peripheral pulse: Pulses that can be assessed in peripheral areas like the extremities.

peripheral vascular resistance (PVR): The resistance to blood moving through the distal vasculature. PVR is an important factor in maintaining normal blood pressure.

peritonitis: Inflammation of the peritoneum—the membrane lining the abdominal cavity (parietal peritoneum) and covering the abdominal organs (visceral peritoneum).

petechial rash: Small, pinpoint reddish dots seen on the surface of the skin resulting from capillary bleeding; often associated with infections like meningitis or disseminated intravascular bleeding.

pH: A measure of the acidity of a solution.

phlebitis: Inflammation of the vein.

phospholipid bilayer: The cell membrane's double layer, consisting of a hydrophilic outer layer composed of phosphate groups, and a hydrophobic inner layer made up of lipids, or fatty acids. It is this structure and composition that allows the cell membrane to have selective permeability.

piercing spike: The hard, sharpened plastic spike on the end of the administration set designed to pierce the sterile membrane of the IV bag.

"piggyback" administration: The addition of a second IV administration set to a primary line via an access port.

plaque: A fatty substance that accumulates within the walls of arteries and can eventually occlude circulation.

pleural lining: The single-cell thick membrane covering the lungs.

pneumatic anti-shock garments (PASG): An inflatable pant that is used to treat shock.

polyuria: The passage of an unusually large volume of urine in a given period; in diabetes, polyuria can result from excreting excess glucose in the urine.

postictal phase: Period following a seizure and lasting between 5 and 30 minutes, characterized by labored respirations and some degree of altered mental status.

postural hypotension: Symptomatic drop in blood pressure related to the patient's body position. Postural hypotension is detected by measuring pulse and blood pressure while the patient is lying supine, sitting up, and standing. An increase in pulse rate and a decrease in blood pressure in any one of these positions is considered a positive sign for postural hypotension.

pressure point: The point where an artery can be compressed against a bone, effectively shutting off flow below the compressed artery.

progressive stage: A stage of shock where fluid losses can be as great as 40%.

prothrombin: One of the initial substrates responsible for clotting cascade activation.

proximal tibial plateau: Anatomical location for intraosseous IV insertion; the flat portion of the tibia located directly below the knee.

psychomotor seizure: A type of seizure characterized by drowsiness, listlessness, or even violence and often associated with a loss of consciousness.

pulmonary edema: A build-up of fluid in the lungs, usually as a result of congestive heart failure.

pulmonary embolus: A blood clot trapped within the pulmonary circulation.

pulse rate: The pressure wave that occurs as each heartbeat causes a surge in the blood circulating through the arteries; the rate at which the heart is contracting. The normal pulse rate in an adult is 60 to 80 beats per minute; for a child, the normal rate is 80 to 100 beats per minute.

pulseless electrical activity (PEA): A cardiac dysrhythmia characterized by the absence of the mechanical pumping function of the heart even though electrical activity is present on a cardiac monitor.

pupillary response: The involuntary response of the pupils to ambient light.

radial pulse: The pulse taken at the radial artery—the major artery in the lower arm, palpable at the wrist on the thumb side.

radiopaque: Invisible on X-rays.

relative contraindication: A situation in which a treatment could have a negative impact, but the benefits of treatment could outweigh the negative impact. Judgment must be used on a case-by-case basis when deciding whether or not to treat in the presence of a relative contraindication.

renin: A potent vasoconstrictor released by the kidneys that constricts the veins in an effort to increase the circulating volume, for example, during shock.

repetitive motor activity: A movement of the body that occurs over and over again, such as lip smacking or pill rolling of the fingers, usually caused by a seizure.

respiratory alkalosis: A metabolic state of alkalosis resulting from excessive losses of carbon dioxide secondary to hyperventilation.

reticular activation system (RAS): The system that is responsible for regulating the conscious state; it consists of the brainstem, pons, medulla, midbrain, hypothalamus, and thalamus.

Rh factor: An additional surface marker on the blood cell. The Rh factor of someone's blood can have grave consequences if incompatible factors are genetically combined.

roller clamp wheel: A device on the administration set tubing that can be rolled across the line to control flow rate into the patient.

rouleaux formation: The stacking of blood cells in the capillary beds. These plugs develop during extreme acidosis and prevent capillary circulation.

saline lock: A special type of IV, also called a buff cap or heparin cap.

SAMPLE history: A key brief history of a patient's condition to determine Signs/symptoms, Allergies, Medications, Pertinent past history, Last oral intake, and Events leading to the illness/injury.

sclerosis: The hardening of a vein from scar tissue after repeated cannulation.

seizure disorder: A syndrome of recurrent seizures that is not due to an underlying metabolic cause.

selective permeability: The ability of the cell membrane to selectively allow compounds into the cell based on the cell's current needs.

sepsis: (1) An infection that has spread to other areas of the body; (2) multiple infections occurring at the same time; (3) reaction to the spilled contents of destroyed cells, as seen with crushed tissue and organs.

septic shock: Shock caused by severe bacterial infection.

serous linings: Single-cell thick membranes found covering organs.

sharps container: A closed, rigid receptacle in which sharp used items such as syringes and scalpels must be discarded.

shock: A condition that develops when the circulatory system is not able to deliver sufficient blood to body organs, resulting in organ failure and eventual death if untreated; also called hypoperfusion.

shock position: The position that has the head and torso (trunk) supine and the lower extremities elevated 8 to 12 inches. This helps to increase blood flow to the brain; also referred to as the modified Trendelenburg's position.

simple partial seizure: A seizure that does not affect consciousness but can affect areas of the brain controlling auditory, motor, or autonomic functions.

skin tenting: The bunching of skin when it is pinched in order to assess for elasticity; this often occurs in dehydrated patients. When the skin of a dehydrated patient is pinched to assess for elasticity, it remains bunched up.

sodium/potassium (Na⁺/K⁺) pump: The mechanism by which the cell brings in two potassium (K^+) ions and releases three sodium (Na^+) ions.

spidery veins: Small veins that weave back and forth; these are a poor choice to start an IV.

standard of care: A uniform level of care that EMTs are expected to provide to all patients.

stroke: A term used to describe an ischemic brain injury, resulting from a sudden loss of blood flow to areas of the brain.

stroke volume: Defined as the amount of blood that the left ventricle can hold during filling.

subdural hematoma: Intracerebral bleeding between the brain and the linings of the brain, most commonly associated with venous bleeding.

surface antigen: A surface marker on the blood cell that identifies circulating immune components as either self or non-self.

sympathetic nervous system: The part of the autonomic nervous system responsible for defensive, compensatory responses; often called the "flight or fight" system.

sympathetic response: Stimulation of the autonomic nervous system's "fight or flight" response.

sympathetic tone: The ability of the sympathetic nervous system to maintain control over the vascular compartment.

syncopal episode: An incidence of fainting or loss of consciousness.

syrup of ipecac: A substance given to induce vomiting.

systemic: Affecting the entire body.

systemic complication: Moderate to severe allergic reaction affecting the systems of the body.

systolic pressure: The pressure created from the contraction and ejection of blood from the left ventricle.

T-cells: The immune cells responsible for remembering antigens and how to destroy them. T-cells are destroyed by HIV.

tachyarrhythmia: Any rapid, non-sinus heart rhythm.

tachycardia: Rapid heart rhythm, more than 100 beats per minute.

tachypnea: Rapid respirations.

tamponade: The application of pressure to a vein to prevent blood flow.

tension pneumothorax: An accumulation of air or gas in the pleural cavity that progressively increases and causes a rise in intrathoracic pressure.

tetanus: A rapidly developing infection that targets the central nervous system. Symptoms include headache, irritability, fever, and ultimately painful muscle spasms that become continuous muscle contractions.

third spacing: The shifting of fluid into the tissues, creating edema.

thoracoabdominal: The anatomical areas of the chest and abdomen.

thrombin: The converted form of prothrombin that begins the clotting cascade.

thrombolytics: A term that refers to a class of drugs designed to re-open occluded arteries associated with acute myocardial infarctions and strokes.

tonic-clonic seizure: A grand mal seizure that features rhythmic back-and-forth motion of an extremity and body stiffness.

tonicity: The osmotic pressure of a solution, based on the relationship between sodium and water inside and outside the cell, that takes advantage of their chemical and osmotic properties to move water to areas of higher sodium concentration.

tort: A civil wrong that can end in a lawsuit even if no criminal act has been committed.

track marks: The visible scars from repeated cannulation of a vein associated with illicit drug use.

transfusion reaction: A potentially life-threatening complication seen during a blood transfusion that occurs when incompatible blood types are introduced.

tricyclics: A class of drugs designed to treat depression; when taken in overdose concentrations, these drugs become cardiotoxic.

tuberculosis: A chronic bacterial disease, caused by *Mycobacterium tuberculosis*, that usually affects the lungs, but can also affect other organs such as the brain and kidneys.

tubule: A section of the kidney where the filtration of wastes, electrolytes, and water is controlled.

unfused cranial plate: The plates of the child's skull anchored to one another by cartilage.

uremia: Excessive levels of urea in the blood.

uremic encephalopathy: Atrophy of cerebral tissue due to the build up of urea from dysfunctioning kidneys.

urticaria: Small spots of generalized itching and/or burning that appear as multiple raised areas on the skin; hives.

Vacutainer: A device that connects to a catheter to assist with blood collection.

varicose veins: A medical condition caused by blood pooling, usually in the legs, resulting from faulty valves in the veins.

vasoconstriction: The narrowing of any blood vessel, especially the veins and arterioles of the skin.

vasodilation: Widening of a blood vessel.

vasovagal reaction: Sudden hypotension and fainting associated with a traumatic or medical event.

venipuncture: The physical puncturing of vein.

venous thrombosis: The development of a stationary blood clot in the venous circulation.

Index

Additional Photo Credits

Chapter 1
Figure 1.1 © Linda Gheen; **Figure 1.4** © Craig Jackson, In the Dark Photography

Chapter 5
Figure 5.2 © Craig Jackson, In the Dark Photography

Chapter 6
Figure 6.7 courtesy of Laerdal Medical Corp.; **Figure 6.13** courtesy of the National EMSC Slideset

Chapter 7
Figure 7.6 courtesy of the American Academy of Orthopaedic Surgeons

Chapter 8
Figure 8.2 courtesy of Ron Dieckmann, MD; **Figure 8.3** © Linda Gheen; **Figure 8.5** courtesy of the National EMSC Slideset; **Figure 8.7** courtesy of Ron Dieckmann, MD